Licensed to Kill

Licensed to Kill

Doctors, the AMA, the FDA and
Pharmasutical company's Greed is Killing You

BY

BARBARA EVERY

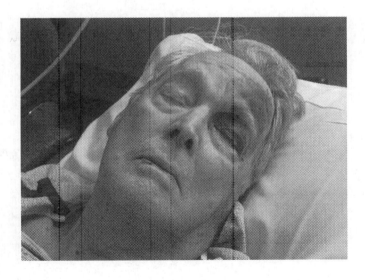

authorHOUSE®

AuthorHouse™
1663 Liberty Drive
Bloomington, IN 47403
www.authorhouse.com
Phone: 1-800-839-8640

Published by AuthorHouse   12/19/2012

ISBN: 978-1-4772-9891-6 (sc)
ISBN: 978-1-4772-9902-9 (e)

Library of Congress Control Number: 2012923459

Preface

In writing this book, I aim to contribute to the education of Americans and to interests in alternative health knowledge. It is not intended to replace MDs or doctor-patient relations. You should always consult a physician if you are sick. If you break an arm or leg, you need a doctor; if you are hurt in an accident, you need a doctor.

Medical education, while detailed, lacks information on nutrition, vitamins, minerals, and herbs. It is my hope that in the near future, this sort of preventative health and alternative health information will be taught to our future doctors.

This lack of any education about natural cures is wrong.

Doctors are supposed to *heal* people and cannot do this if their education includes only one aspect of the healing equation. Unfortunately, *medical* school is just what the name implies. Were doctors to have access to information on both medicine and natural healing, more people would be able to find good health. Then, we could change the name of *medical* schools to *health* schools.

No one appears to even be trying to break the stronghold the pharmaceutical industry has on medical schools, the Food and Drug Administration (FDA), the American Medical Association (AMA), doctors, advertising and media companies, and, unfortunately, many politicians. Someone or some organization needs to take the challenge, or the present situation of increasing illness, disease, and unnatural death will be exacerbated. So, with this book, I wish to do my part to try to make more of the population aware of the very precarious relationship among individuals, our health, and the medical industry.

Acknowledgments

I dedicate this book to my family and to everyone who seeks real cures and good health through natural, God-given, better means like nutrition, herbs, vitamins, and minerals. This book is also dedicated to all people that are concerned that our medical schools teach only drugs (poisons) and surgical techniques, and who hope that in the near future, doctors' educations will include the best natural cures—prevention and nutrition.

I give special thanks to my husband, for his research and editing were of vital importance in the development of this book. I am grateful that he allowed me to use his pictures and the story of his adverse reactions to prescription drugs and the American Heart Association (AHA) diet.

Miracles Do Happen!

This book is written under the protection of the First Amendment of the Constitution of the United States of America—the freedom of speech!

I do not have any license, so I can't lose one. I do not have an office, so cannot be closed down. I do not sell anything, so there is no inventory to confiscate.

There are many organizations that may object to what I write, in particular pharmaceutical companies, the AMA, and the FDA (our Government), even though the facts and figures have been obtained from very reliable sources of information. Qualified alternative doctors, homeopaths, scientists and others have gone on their own to gain important knowledge on nutrition, vitamins, minerals and herbs for proven, natural, God-given cures!

Table of Contents

Chapter One: Causes of Death 1

Chapter Two: Follow the Money 11

Chapter Three: A Few of the Facts 19

Chapter Four: Are We Still in the Dark Ages? 81

Chapter Five: You Are What You Eat!. 91

Chapter Six: Obesity and Diet 99

Chapter Seven: Colloidal Silver and Hydrogen Peroxide. 109

Chapter Eight: A Merry Heart—Another Natural Cure 113

Chapter Nine: Here we go Again! 121

Chapter Ten: Government *of* the People? 127

Chapter Eleven: Cutting Off Their Nose to Spite

                  Their Face or Shooting Themselves

                  in the Foot! 151

Chapter One

CAUSES OF DEATH

The number one cause of death isn't heart disease or cancer—it isn't vehicular accidents. According to a booklet from Health Central Hospital (A Florida hospital in Ocoee), "Medical errors are a leading cause of Death in the United States." And according to Dr. Bruce West founder of *Health Alert News in* (Aug.-Sept 2011 page 1), "Medical treatments cause more deaths than any disease."

Heart disease is listed as the number one cause of death and cancer listed as the second most-prevalent cause of death. However with drugs, surgery, and medical treatments (and any resulting medical errors) used as treatment for both of these conditions, as well as innumerable other health conditions, it isn't difficult to realize what the true cause of the most deaths really is!

According to *The Inquisitor,* some "statistics which were taken in 2009 shows that 37,485 people died in traffic related accidents while 36,284 people died from drug related activities in one year period."[1] Other statistics point to a general problem in the relationship between ailments and treatments:

106,000 patients are killed every year by prescription drugs;
1 in 4 patients suffer from prescription drug's side effects;
1,000,000 deaths each year are caused by medical care;

1

20,000,000 unnecessary antibiotics are prescribed every year;
7,500,000 surgeries and medical procedures are performed annually that are not needed; and
2,500,000 patients are seriously injured every year by prescription drugs.

Ninety-five percent of the three billion prescriptions issued annually are handwritten, which can lead to undocumented mistakes! Federal officials have not yet approved of electronic prescriptions to avoid these mistakes. [3]

Simvastatin is only one component of the "wonder drugs" (the statins). The list goes on and on and continues to grow.

I wonder how the pharmaceutical companies, the Federal Drug Administration—FDA, Federal Trade Commission—FTC, and American Medical Association—AMA became all-powerful. Doctors can actually lose their license if they incorporate natural cures, herbs, vitamins and minerals into their practice. Their offices can be raided with armed people wearing government badges; they can seize all records and whatever else they choose. I will address these raids more specifically in chapter ten, where I detail real cases of doctors' offices being raided and some doctors losing their licenses.

How did these institutions become all-powerful? Why do medical schools rarely include education for doctors on diet and nutrition? Why do future doctors accept educations that lack in information on diet and nutrition? Didn't their mothers ever tell them anything about eating good foods so they would grow up strong and healthy? Haven't we all heard from our mothers while growing up, "You are what you eat!"?

The answer to all of these questions is quite easy to understand: money.

How many Americans, including our government officials, know that the doctors in eight years of medical school do not receive information on nutrition, vitamins, herbs, or minerals? Some doctors may get only a few hours of education about infant nutrition.

Doctors are only taught (brainwashed) about drugs (prescriptions) and surgery. That's the way the AMA, big pharmaceutical companies, the FDA, and the FTC want it! However, it isn't really appropriate to blame the doctors for this imbalanced knowledge and training; it is a result of the power of the afore-mentioned groups. Most of us admire our doctors, but unfortunately rely on them to cure all of our ailments. Doctors can only know what to do for us based on the only information (misinformation) they have been taught—writing prescriptions or performing surgeries.

Chiropractors actually receive more hours of nutrition, vitamins and prescription drug education during their eight years of study than MDs. Chiropractors also obtain more information on nutrition, vitamins, and minerals. The chiropractor who treated my husband and me in Florida did not have any health insurance. When asked why, he responded, "Why would I need any?"

We all seem to have bought into "big pharma's" ongoing propaganda "hook, line, and sinker." And you know what happens to every fish that takes the bait—they are goners! It looks like the same thing is happening to people—thousands continue to die from prescription drugs (the bait). Disregard your health and it will soon be gone.

I am writing this book because of the severity of the above facts and because I hope that my voice may contribute to a solution. It is my hope that the travesty of doctors not getting any information on nutrition in eight years of (medical) training can be revised, and information on real, God-given, natural cures can also be included!

We became driven to study as much as possible through books, health newsletters, and whatever sources we can find on natural healing. Much of this knowledge has taken others (alternative doctors and scientists) years to study and prove.

We now have more information on nutrition than most AMA doctors. And at the ages of eighty and eight-two, we have a wealth of experiences to draw upon. (It took us a lot of years to get this old—even several decades!)

Due to having the same or similar information from several sources, I may not be giving credit to all specific persons, books,

Newsletters, etc. each time because this information has been obtained from more than one origin of knowledge.

Due to irrefutable scientific studies as noted through out this book[4] and research, (and my own anecdotal experiences and studies), a lack of certain vitamins and minerals are not only the cause of all illnesses, they are also the cure! It has been proven that no degenerative diseases have ever been cured by pharmaceutical drugs. Prescription drugs are just a cover up, and not a cure! These drugs address only the symptoms of illness, not the root cause.

It has also been proven that God's nutritional vitamins, herbs and minerals have erased (cured) illnesses by eliminating the cause, which is caused by a Lack of proper nutrition.

The Book of Mormon: Another Testimony of Jesus Christ[5] states in Alma 46:40 (regarding the many wars and deaths), " . . . not so much so with fevers, because of the excellent qualities of plants and roots which God had prepared to remove the cause of disease, to which men were subject by the nature of the climate."

Do any of us have bodies that are low on any drugs (Poisons)? If you don't believe drugs are poisons, just read some of the side effects that come with all prescriptions. Many, or most all, also list death as a possible side effect. Isn't this just what poisons do? Our bodies are not created with any prescription and over the counter drugs!

The Webster's New Collegiate Dictionary[6] defines poison as, "Any substance which kills or injures when introduced into a living organism; that which has an evil influence on health or moral purity; having a deadly or injurious quality." It might instead be more appropriate to examine on which vitamins and minerals we might be low. It has been found by the alternative health doctors and scientist that many health problems are the result of a deficiency of various vitamins and minerals, not a deficiency of medicines (drugs or poisons).

Degenerative diseases are the result of a lack of certain nutrients. Therefore, the cure for degenerative diseases is to address the lack of these nutrients. Consider polio and the polio vaccine. Polio is a virus. A vaccine has been developed and has stopped the spread of polio, but there is no cure for polio once a person is infected with the disease.

At the height of the polio epidemic in 1949, Dr. Frederick Klenner treated sixty polio victims in his office and in the emergency room at the hospital where he practiced. He cured all sixty patients with large, intravenous doses of vitamin C in a matter of days. None of the sixty experienced any residual side effects at any time. That's a one hundred percent cure—it doesn't get any better! [7]

Dr. Klenner spoke about his vitamin "C" cure at an AMA meeting, but it never left the room! Did the doctors present think it was too simple? Did they find it too good to be true? Did they think that Dr. Klenner should have used drugs instead or that he was lying? Perhaps, instead, they kept the solution secret because it didn't hold enough potential for generating revenue.

How many polio victims did the "iron lung" cure?

If you are one of the doubters who thinks this is too good or simple to be true, then you can check it out on Medline, the database of the National Library of Medicine. This publicly accessible resource is also where doctors learn about current research. Medline contains over 11,000,000 citations and author abstracts from over 4,000 biomedical journals from all over the world. Dr. Klenner has conducted other research, particularly with vitamin C, for diseases other than polio.

My husband and I have a friend who had polio as a child and now has a severe limp. He requires a special, cane-like device with arm braces for support in order to walk. He has since heard about Dr. Klenner and wished the doctors that treated him had known about the vitamin C treatment. But he was one of the more fortunate polio cases—he is still alive and functional.

We must broaden our approach to health to include nutritional information. If it doesn't change, our very lives are at stake; there will continue to be increasing illness, disease, and untimely death.

Often upon graduation from medical school, new doctors may receive gifts from the pharmaceutical companies. Some aggressive pharmaceutical sales representatives give practicing doctors gifts for prescribing drugs. Doctors can even receive money for prescribing prescription drugs. Are we to believe these gifts are given to graduating doctors and practicing doctors because they are so well-liked? Or are these gifts motivated by money?

The forms that patients have to fill out in the doctor's offices and the questions doctors rarely ask about nutritional information.

Have you ever had a doctor ask you about your diet?

Have you ever had a doctor ask you about what vitamins you were taking?

Has a doctor ever even suggested you should be taking certain vitamins?

Have you ever had a doctor ask you about what drugs you were taking? (I sure have—every time!)

Have any of the forms (sometimes several pages) you have to fill out at the doctor's office asked for a list of the vitamins and minerals you are taking?

Have these forms requested a list of the drugs you take? I have been in a doctor's office and have heard some patients ask for more paper in order to list all of the drugs they are taking!

Has a doctor ever given you an additional prescription because of the side effects of a prescription you were already taking?

One of the doctors I saw regularly added another prescription every time I went in, until I had accumulated six different prescriptions. I was not taking any medicines when I first went to him. He also told me that buying vitamins is a waste of money and that "All vitamins do is give you expensive urine." As a result of this interaction I changed to another Doctor and am now back to no prescriptions. I feel much better, even though I am several years older now!

My husband and I have another friend who takes over a dozen different prescriptions that he says he *needs* because of a heart condition. He takes certain medications in the morning and the rest of them in the evening. He has to keep them straight, because if he should get them mixed up, and take too many of any one of them, there could be some very serious side effects!

I imagine "big pharma" would like to have a lot more prescription takers like these! It equals money and more money for them! Many of these people are told they will need to take all these medications for the rest of their lives, which means "big pharma" will continue collecting money until—you guessed it—death.

Are you aware that some doctors will actually continue to prescribe drugs even though the drugs have been proven useless or even dangerous?

What do the doctors have to lose? The drug companies cannot be sued—the warnings were given to you when you got the prescriptions

More people die from drugs (prescription and over-the-counter), doctors' mistakes, pharmacy errors, hospital stays, and hospital visits than from any other causes of death! Perhaps the AMA should be called American *Murder* Association or the FDA should be called the Federal *Death* Administration.

How many people do you know that do not go to a doctor? How many people do you know that do not take some kind of prescription, and on a regular basis? I suspect you could count them on one hand.

People often do pick up viruses, diseases and so on from the hospitals, even though it might just be a short visit to a friend or relative. After all, the hospitals are full of people with all kinds of illnesses. People don't typically visit hospitals when they are well. Some strains of viruses are so potent that they have grown resistant to antibiotics. Doctor's offices are also filled with sick people

Taking what seems to be harmless, over the counter drugs, like cold or allergy medicine or pain relievers, has caused some really big problems for even healthy people.

Aspirin, ibuprofen, and other popular pain relievers contain acetaminophen, which can cause acute liver damage. Approximately 26,000 people are hospitalized yearly for using these drugs, with liver failure. The ingredient, acetaminophen, is used in over one hundred different over-the-counter cold, insomnia, allergy, and other remedies.[8]

You may feel short term relief while using these pain killers, but you could also experience some very nasty side effects later on. They can cause serious stomach bleeding, for example. There are some 20,000 deaths per year resulting from these easy to get, over-the-counter, drugs.

Salicylates[9]—the pain-killing ingredient found in aspirins—is also found in almonds! Wouldn't you rather enjoy a small handful of almonds than risk aspirin's dangerous side effects? We can all be "nutty" and safe.

There are an enormous number of people taking over-the-counter medicines for upset stomach, heartburn, acid reflux, etc. These easily-available medications (mostly acid reducers) do give some temporary relief, but can cause harmful side effects with long-term use. Our bodies should basically be slightly alkaline although the stomach does have a certain amount acid. It requires acid to digest food, so completely reducing the acid is not the solution. As we age, the stomach acid is naturally reduced[10].

Whenever either my husband and I might have an upset stomach or possible heartburn, we just take a small sip or two of vinegar (acid). This restores the pH balance to the stomach. We are not necessarily fans of the taste of vinegar, but we do prefer the apple cider vinegar to regular white vinegar. Peppermint can also help relieve an irritable bowel problem.

I have also heard that some people put a bit of salt (a good sea salt) on their tongue for stomach problems. My husband and I have tried this and feel that it works great, too! It is certainly better than any antacids that are consumed by the general public to the tune of several millions of dollars yearly!

We have heard that other people who are bothered with acid reflux disease take a spoonful of sauerkraut. This approach is said to be effective when the sauerkraut is taken before each meal. Perhaps the vinegar or the salt in the sauerkraut have the same effect on the stomach's pH as taking those foods directly. Vinegar is also proven to be an aid in weight loss, among myriad other household uses.

Doctors continue to write prescriptions that are killing us slowly because they don't know any better. This is all they have been taught. Take a look in any medical journal—the ones doctors read to keep up on the latest and newest developed information. This "news" is not only funded by the pharmaceutical industry but it is also written by them. Some may be called "ads," but others are labeled "scientific research"! (Yeah, right.)

We need to have doctors to be concerned with the practical consequences of both drugs and nutrition, so we can have the best of both worlds.

1   "The One Minute Cure" by Madison Cavanaugh, published by Think Outside the Book Publishing, Inc, page 17

2   "Bottom Line Books" brochure Spring 2011 issue page 3)

3   (Parade Magazine, Jan. 8, 2008

4   "The FDA Suppression of Cures" by Robert R. Barefoot copyright 2006 ww.BarefootCureAmerica.com
"Curing the Incurable" by Thomas E. Levy, MD, JD copyright 2002 by LivOn Books

5   "The Book of Mormon-Another Testament of Jesus Christ" First published in March 1830 Page 325

6   "The Webster's New Collegiate Dictionary" Copyright 1956 page?????)

7   http://www.doctoryourself.com/klennerbio.html

8   "Ultimate Healing" by Dr. Anne Larson, MD published by Bottom Line Books 2011—Page 127

9   "2-Day Migraine Cured in Minutes" by Joan Wilen and Lydia Wilen published by Bottom Line Books Fall 2007—Page 8

10 On FOX News (TV) on 9-16-2011, "Actos is linked to bladder cancer"!

Chapter Two

FOLLOW THE MONEY

You can hardly turn around without seeing or hearing about a new, "must-have" drug about which you should "talk to your doctor." Most newspaper, magazine, radio, and television ads are loaded with commercials that reflect favorably on drugs. They emphasize all the so-called wonders the drugs are supposed to do for you, only touch on some of the side effects [1], while showing people doing pleasurable activities. This makes it difficult for the viewer, listener, or reader to pay attention to the information on side effects, even when it is as serious of "thoughts of suicide" or "death." You know the saying, "One picture is worth a thousand words!" People see the picture but have a more difficult time processing the language.

Since statin drugs came on the scene, hospitalizations for heart failure have increased more than 130 percent! [2]

These widely-prescribed statin drugs (poisons) with many dangerous side effects (from heartburn to fatalities) brought in more than fourteen billion dollars in 2010 alone! These drugs are being prescribed more and more frequently, which means they will continue to bring in more and more money to the drug companies. And where does all this money come from? Us! Drug companies can't just print more money like our government does. And in fact, they don't need to because they're already making billions off of the population at large.

Even worse, the side effects of these drugs often contribute to or worsen exactly what they are supposed to be helping or curing.

Celebrex, for instance, has TV ads that feature elderly people in the background stretching, bending, and moving about freely. What's in motion tends to stay in motion. Many of the elderly who have been given a prescription for this wonder drug (poison) say they felt much worse after taking it.

Celebrex is still on the market, although Vioxx has fortunately been taken off because of too many drug-related deaths. Osteoporosis, the "silent disease," is said to affect one-half of women over fifty years of age, and one-fourth of men. What is happening to these people that have been prescribed medications for this problem? They continue to experience broken bones, particularly hip fractures.

And one-fourth of patients with hip fractures die within a year of complications. Others who were seemingly healthy prior to their fractures, require long term care, which is known to be expensive.

How many years have we been told we should take Tylenol (acetaminophen) because it was purported to be much safer than any other pain killers? It has now been proven[3] that this wonder-drug causes liver damage and cancer. As a result, some types of acetaminophen are being called off the market. But just think about all the money that Tylenol brought in over all these years before the (partial) recall! Even worse than the money are the illnesses and disasters that Tylenol has caused over all the years it has been on the market!

Many dentists are refusing to take patients that are taking Fosamax because it is causing "bone rot" or the deterioration of the jaw bone. On June 8, 2011, many news stations featured a Zocor warning. If you take eighty milligrams you are going to have problems! The FDA issued this warning: "The U.S. Food and Drug Administration (FDA) is recommending limiting the use of the highest approved dose of the cholesterol-lowering medication, simvastatin (80 mg) because of **increased risk of muscle damage**.

Simvastatin 80 mg should be used only in patients who have been taking this dose for 12 months or more without evidence of muscle injury (myopathy). Simvastatin 80 mg should not be started in new patients, including patients already taking lower doses of the drug. In addition to these new limitations, FDA is requiring changes to the simvastatin label to add new contraindications (should not be used with certain medications) and dose limitations for using simvastatin with certain medicines."[4][5]

Traveling salespeople, truck drivers, students studying late at night, and other ordinary folks buy over-the-counter stimulants to the tune of 100 billion dollars per year to boost their energy.

One fairly recent addition to this market, Five Hour Energy, boasts that it will give you five hours of great energy from its 1.93-ounce container. It is sold in a variety of stores—grocery stores, drug stores, and convenience stores, among others. It has a robust television ad campaign, especially during sports programming. This is not cheap advertising. When you read the ingredients listed, the first ingredient (and therefore the most prevalent) named is water. This is mighty expensive water! There are also a couple of preservatives like sodium benzoate. Five Hour Energy used to advertise no calories, but more recent ads claim four calories alongside a picture of an avocado, a piece of broccoli and a banana coming out of the container. How small of an amount of these three items would it take to get only four calories? Caffeine is another so-called energy booster. Coffee also has caffeine and thein, both of which are poisonous alkaloids when present in large enough quantities. The price for this flavored water is almost three dollars per container.

Like the old saying goes, "There's a sucker born every minute."

"Brain fog" or a clouding of the consciousness is being caused by some of the top prescribed dementia drugs. These drugs are being given out almost like candy in many nursing homes. Many of these drugs are no more effective than a placebo (and maybe a placebo would be better[6])! All of these brain fog medications have made the drug companies more big fortunes. Even if the medicine isn't legitimate, the money brought in from it is. Nursing homes are a golden goose for pharmaceutical companies.

One of the dementia cases that I read about, in more than one health newsletters, involved a husband whose dementia was so bad he couldn't recognize any of his family and didn't even know his own name[7]. His brain fog was so bad he couldn't even remember how to use a spoon and had to be fed. He, of course, lost his job—which was quite technical and used to give him a lot of pleasure. He could do complicated math in his head, would take apart computers and repair them, could fix just about anything, and had a quick wit. With such severe dementia, he also started wandering and getting lost. It was causing his wife and family considerable problems, to say the least.

His wife (Dr. Mary N.) got on the internet and discovered there was a natural medicine, Keyasyn, with which people were having great results for the treatment of dementia. The main ingredient was coconut oil. She purchased coconut oil at a local health food store and began giving it to her husband. His brain fog began improving almost immediately. After some time he was so improved that he was even able to go back to work! If he happens to forget to take the coconut oil, signs of the dementia begin to return until he is able to take it again.

Coconut oil is not only cheaper, but has no side effects and you do not need a prescription in order to get it. I have seen coconut oil in grocery stores lately. It is called an oil, but exists in a solid consistency below seventy-five degrees and as an oil above seventy-seven degrees. Coconut oil is good in cooking, from baking to frying.

This is most certainly a lot healthier than any brain fog drugs that are not only expensive, but require a doctor's written prescription in order to be obtained. Over 3,000 Alzheimer's patients have been significantly helped with a natural botanical extract. This extract not only stops the decline of mental function and memory, but it can even improve memory! Those patients who took the extract did seven times better than those that did not in memory retention. It is made of daffodils, snowdrops, spider lilies, and other plants. Just like in the springtime when these flowers bloom, this extract gives new life to Alzheimer's patients.

The drugs from the pharmaceutical industry lose their effectiveness within a short time, but these botanical wonders keep on working. In five separate studies on thousands of Alzheimer's patients in Belgium this extract worked every single time.

Sorry drug companies and funeral parlors, there's no money here for you!

How often are we now hearing on the news that a drug is being recalled, because of the great number of deaths resulting from the users? One of the drugs for diabetes was recalled after almost 400 people died of liver failure! An FDA warning: [5-18-2011] The U.S. Food and Drug Administration (FDA) is informing the public of new restrictions to the prescribing and use of rosiglitazone-containing medicines. These medicines to treat type II diabetes are sold under the names Avandia, Avandamet, and Avandaryl. Healthcare providers and patients must enroll in a special program in order to prescribe and receive these drugs.

The new restrictions are part of a Risk Evaluation and Mitigation Strategy (REMS)—a program FDA may require to manage serious risks of marketed drugs. The restrictions are based on data that suggested an elevated risk of heart attacks in patients treated with rosiglitazone. The decision to restrict access to rosiglitazone medicines was made on September 23, 2010.

FDA has modified the REMS for Avandamet and Avandaryl because previously, the REMS consisted of only a Medication Guide. The REMS, which now includes a restricted access and distribution program, applies to all three rosiglitazone products.[8] An October 2011 Avandia warning cautioned that the drug can cause "heart attack, stroke, other heart problems, and death." The deaths caused by these drugs (poisons) number in the hundreds and often thousands before the drug can be considered for a recall. The FDA admitted that Vioxx killed over 25,000 people before it was taken off the market![9] This is a serious and dangerous state of affairs to our very precious lives and an outrage that needs to be stopped now.

Consider the money that drug companies have made from these hundreds (sometimes thousands) of people prior to their demise. Why recall a gold mine before you have to? Maybe this is why the doctor's business is called "a practice"! And who are the doctor's practicing on? Us, the patients!

One rarely, if ever, reads or hears about any vitamins, minerals, or herbs being taken off the market, or even warnings of serious side effects. These are natural God-given cures that He has provided for our health and use.

Previously, when I mention "wishful thinking" as motivation for writing this book, I am talking about the challenge of getting powerful drug companies to change their policies. This is a different sort of "Golden Rule" for the Pharmaceutical companies—they sure make a lot of gold, and therefore, they make all the rules! I also call this the "Follow the Money Rule." Newspaper, magazine, radio, and television ads bring in the most money for these companies. It's the money, money, money!

At least twenty years ago, when my husband and I first had a business of our own, we called a nationally-known magazine to inquire about placing a one-page advertisement. Even at this time it cost several thousand dollars for just a single-page ad. If I remember correctly, It was over $25,000. I can't imagine what the cost would be now! The ads for prescription drugs from various sources comprise twenty-five percent of all advertising. Here are a few examples:

In the January 2011 issue of *Women's Day* magazine there were seven ads for drugs that took a lot more than seven pages, because of the long list of information (mainly side effects) that accompanied them. The ads included such medications as Orencia (abatacept, two pages); Lyrica (pregabalin, two pages; Vimovo (naproxen/esomeprazole magnesium, three pages); Gardasil (Human Papillomavirus Quadrivalent two pages); Simponi (golimumab, four pages); Seroquel (quetiapine, four pages); and Cimzia (certolizumab pegol two pages) of the ads totaled nineteen pages. If one page cost several thousands of dollars, this pharmaceutical spread certainly adds up to a lot of advertising revenue for the magazine!

The same Magazine also had two ads for vitamins—Vitamin D3 (5000 IU, one page) and Mega Red (5000 IU, one page). Because these vitamins have of no side effects, their advertisements only required pages, and therefore there is nowhere near as much advertising money (profits) per product!

In the July 2011 issue of *Better Homes and Gardens* [11] there were ads for Humira (adalimumab, four pages);Reclast (zoledronic acid, three pages); Vimovo (naproxen esomeprazol magnesium, two pages). Gardasil (Human Paillomvirus Quadracalent two pages), and Exelon Patch (three pages). That totals fourteen pages on drugs and side effects. At several thousands of dollars per page that adds up to a heck of a lot of "dough"! There were no ads for Vitamins.

It doesn't take a math genius to see why magazines, radio stations, television stations, newspapers, billboards, websites and other venues would even consider *not* accepting ads for drugs. "big pharma" brings them their biggest profits!

In the ads for the drugs the scientific names are like mumbo-jumbo to many of us. We couldn't even begin to pronounce most of these technical names, and what they mean in terms of ingredients is really foreign. Even my new computer doesn't recognize them! Most of us are familiar with terms of IU (International Units) and mg (milligrams) used for most vitamins and minerals. By the way, 20 mg equal 1,000,000 IUs. There are 1,000 mg in a gram (g), and 28.57 g in an ounce.

The pharmaceutical companies won't give us the natural cures for any of life-threatening diseases because there is no money in it for them. They can try as they might, to duplicate a natural cure with drugs, but cannot be nearly as effective as natural cures. Even if the drug companies can come up with something similar, they can charge whatever they choose, which could be in the billions annually! According to the National Academy of Sciences, it generally takes seventeen years for so-called important research to reach hospitals and doctors. Natural cures are available *now* and more and more cures found in nature are continually being discovered and offered to us almost immediately.

[1] Example of this with print advertising: "Woman's Day" magazine July 2011. advertisement on Page 58-61—Page 59—"These are not all of the possible side effects with HUMERA. For more information, talk to your health care provider.

[2] "Health and Healing" brochure by Dr. Julian Whitaker MD, Summer 2011, page 3

[3] "Ultimate Healing" by Dr. Anne Larson, MD. Bottom Line Books Page 127

[4] http://www.fda.gov/Drugs/DrugSafety/ucm256581.htm

[5] Fox News Channel June 8, 2011

[6] Bottom Line Books page 9—Brochure published summer 2011 citing an article in the New England Journal or Medicine

[7] "Real Cures" Newsletter by Dr. Frank Shallenberger June 2011 Pages 1-5

[8] http://www.fda.gov/Drugs/DrugSafety/ucm255005.htm

[9] http://www.techdirt.com/articles/20120625/19574119473/protected-to-death-how-medical-privacy-laws-helped-kill-25000-people.shtml

[10] "Woman's Day" January 2011

[11] "Better Homes and Gardens" July 2011

Chapter Three

A FEW OF THE FACTS

If the radio and TV raves about a remedy with great enthusiasm and people are passionately talking about it, it is probably a myth and should be avoided.

For Instance, last year (2010) crystal meth was cited as a wonder drug for colds and flu cure and prevention. Like my husband and I, you probably didn't know, or even consider, to ask what ingredients are in crystal meth. It includes:

Cold medication
Drano
Brake fluid
Hydrochloric acid
Sodium Hydroxide

I obtained this information from a chiropractor's bulletin board in Florida. [1] If you are like me, you wouldn't want any of this stuff in your body! Our bodies are certainly not naturally lacking in any of it! It is most harmful and damaging to out bodies—It may be OK for toilets, sinks and cars.

Were you aware that the blood thinners, like Coumadin or Warfarin,) that doctors often prescribe for people (often a life sentence) are drugs made from the same ingredients that are in rat poison and can have some very grievous side effects? If these chemicals kill rats, what will they do to people?

Blood thinners are most often prescribed to people with heart problems. Since Heart Disease is said to be the number one cause of death, this makes for an enormous number of prescriptions! There are vitamins that are equally good blood thinners and, surprise, cause no side effects. Vitamin E is only one of them. Drinking more water also helps.

Some research shows that organic mineral iodine and Vitamins E and B complexes are a good way to treat people with a heart rhythm problem. (Read more about iodine in chapter nine, "Here We Go Again.") I have also heard that a vitamin G is good for this problem, but I am not familiar with it. For over a hundred years, Iodine has been used for treating people with irregular heartbeat, though not by the strict AMA doctors. Top-grade "Iosol" iodine is available from larger health food stores or from the retailers listed below:

Mountain Home Nutritionals
700 Indian Springs Drive
Lancaster, PA. 17601
Phone 1-800-888-1415
Zerbos
34164 Plymouth Road
Livonia, Michigan 48150
734-427-3144

Iosol brand has also been recommended by some of the doctors in the health news letters that we receive. It comes in a one-ounce bottle (with an eye dropper lid) for approximately $18. You will only need one or two drops for general maintenance. Each bottle contains over 600 drops, so it goes a long way. Iodine could easily be called the mineral of many miracles, because it can be used to cure even more than a-Fib (atrial fibrillation).

There was a physician who traveled from village to village in Africa for thirty years and drank contaminated water, but never once got sick! Because he always put two or three drops of Iodine in the water a few minutes before he drank it[2]. It's a good thing to have with you especially when you travel and are unsure of any water. Remember most towns in the United States add chemicals to their water systems. In cases of fibrocystic breast disease, six to eight drops in a few ounces of water taken daily can cure it in three to six months. Iodine can also be used to treat bladder infections and clogged arteries. If you have trouble with gas when consuming products made with beans, add a few drops of Iodine when preparing the recipe.

Not only is Iodine good for our insides, but great for many uses on our outer parts. For hemorrhoids, mix one-half ounce of flaxseed oil with ten drops of iodine and it works almost overnight. Iodine can also be used to treat toenail fungus, infected hangnails, pimples, cold sores, and many other conditions!

SSKI (a saturated solution of potassium iodide) is another form of Iodine. SSKI can be obtained in some compounding pharmacies without a prescription, some health food stores, or online. Contact the International Academy of Compounding Pharmacists (800-927-4227) or www.iacprx.org for additional information.

Magnesium is another nearly magical mineral. It is needed by every cell, tissue, and organ. Most people don't get enough magnesium and most doctors don't know about it's great worth. It combats high blood pressure (hypertension), heart disease, stroke, memory loss, osteoporosis, and diabetes. It would be difficult to get too much magnesium.

My husband and I take three magnesium tablets each day at morning, noon, and evening. The only side effects you might have are if you are not getting enough magnesium, such as the ones listed above. Magnesium is inexpensive and readily available.

CoQ10 (coenzyme Q10) is another needed nutrient that carries power to you cells. Statins (again) block this fuel that is needed by every organ in your body, including your heart (and other muscles) and your brain. Statins have put many people in nursing homes with dementia, but most doctors refuse to make the connection. They were only trying to reduce the patient's cholesterol or treat his or her heart problem, right?

There is no study that can show any benefits derived from a statin drug [3]. So who *needs* a statin drug? And why would they need it? Many of the wonder drugs that are pushed on people by doctors that have been told by the pill peddlers about the drug's supposed cures before they have been fully tested!

Because of all the harmful ingredients that are now being included in medications, it is more important than ever to read and inquire about the ingredients that are in what we buy or in what is prescribed for us.

Food labels are also very important to read. Our foods are being laced with chemicals, such as the so-called preservatives used to lengthen their shelf life. Farmers are spraying their crops with chemicals. Big commercial agricultural producers are also doing a lot of genetic engineering to produce more and larger yields. These could be labeled "fake foods," as they contain very few (if any) nutrients. None of this is done for our good; it is for more profit.

Conversely, it is also important to beware of the word "natural" as used on many food products. Sugar is a natural food and is contained in many of the foods labeled "natural." Several peanut butter brands are labeled "natural," for example. Smucker's is the only brand that we have found in grocery stores that does not contain sugar, but just peanuts.

Along the same lines, poison ivy is also "natural" and so is nightshade! Nightshade is an attractive vine with very small, attractive purple flowers. Later in the season the blossoms are replaced with green berries that finally turn bright red. The berries look tempting to eat, but are very poisonous and there is no known antidote to them! This poisonous plant grows in several states throughout America.)

These plants, naturally, will not be put in our foods. I just wanted to emphasize how misleading the word "natural" can be.

The Pharmaceutical companies are going to continue to concoct more and more drugs, with increasingly serious side effects, including "thoughts of suicide" and "death"—all because of the billions of dollars they bring in!

For instance, one giant pharmaceutical company, AstraZeneca, receives tens of billions of dollars for their statin drug Crestor—the only drug approved by the FDA (what a present this was!) to reduce the risk of a heart attack. But, does it really do this?

There is one death from a heart attack every 52 seconds in the United States.[4] That's about 600,000 heart related deaths yearly!

Let's take former President Bill Clinton, for example. He had bypass surgery in 2004. If it was a cure, why did he have coronary stents put in during 2010? He required further treatment even after he was supposed to be doing "everything right!" So it appears that President Clinton's bypass surgery certainly was not a cure.

Then there is Dick Cheney. It is said, that he has taken statin drugs for decades.[5] These wonder drugs have not prevented him from additional heart attacks. As a matter of fact, he has had them in 1978, 1984, 1988, 2000, and still again in 2010. In 2001 doctors even implanted a pacemaker to control his heart rhythm. Again in 2008, he underwent another procedure to repair his heart to a normal rhythm. With all of this medical attention, why did Dick Cheney experience yet another heart attack in 2010? Would you call all these drugs and surgeries a cure for Mr. Cheney's heart problems? It certainly does not appear that all these procedures were much help at all.

These are the famous people that we all know about, but there are thousand (actually millions) of others that we don't know about and won't hear about, who have had repeated heart procedures.

Certainly no doctor ever told Dick Cheney, or any other heart patient, about the effects of iodine, mentioned earlier. The doctors also do not recommend CoQ10, or soy lecithin granules (to clean arteries), magnesium, or any other vitamins and minerals. Not only does magnesium keep your arteries from cramping, but it prevents heart muscle spasms.

Most people with hypertension (high blood pressure) are prescribed dangerous drugs by their well-intentioned doctors (from what they learned in medical schools). The side effects of the drugs can often be even worse than the disorder itself. There are also natural cures for high blood pressure, like the beet, which will be discussed later in this chapter.

Pharmaceutical companies can claim that their drugs will do whatever they choose to say the drugs will do! However, the list of the different side effects that these drugs can cause is nearly endless, including "thoughts of Suicide" and "death"!

Many of the medications that feature "thoughts of suicide" and "violent actions" as side effects are being prescribed to teenagers and people experiencing depression. Drugs that treat dementia and high blood pressure have similar side effects and are prescribed widely.

At one time, I was prescribed a drug to lower my blood pressure. When the blood pressure remained elevated, my doctor simply prescribed a higher dosage. I also had a rash around my eyes that I couldn't get rid of. I tried to determine whether I was eating anything different. I completely changed all my makeup. With the increased dosage, however, the rash worsened. For some reason, I never associated the rash with the medicine! If I would have read the side effects I would have known the cause. One of the side effects listed was "rash", along with several others. Obviously, I was allergic to it! When I stopped the medicine, not only did the rash go away, but my high blood pressure was also gone! The original high blood pressure was likely a result of simply being in the doctor's office. There is even a name for it, "white coat high blood pressure."

The FDA

Our own federal government is partly responsible for a lack of information about natural remedies. The FDA actually forbids vitamin and mineral suppliers to put on their labels or in their catalogs, any of the healthful benefits or any information about what these vitamins, minerals, or supplements, can do for you! That is, unless the FDA is paid a great amount of money (in the range of $250,000,000) for "approval." [6][7] Because foods, vitamins, minerals and herbs cannot be patented, none of the manufacturers of these natural items can make enough money from them to pay for federal approval. That's right, it's the money again!

Is this a level playing field?

The AMA, the FDA, the pharmaceutical Industry, and strict AMA Doctors don't know about the many natural cures! And the medical schools don't know about them either. What's even worse, these people and organizations don't even want to know about them!

As reported in the Associated Press, "There is no cure for coronary artery disease." Cardiologist have also said they don't have a cure and that patients have to return time and time again for a so-called tune-ups or another treatment, which results in more and more surgery and, of course, more and more money. Drug companies have made fortunes from doctors prescribing cholesterol-lowering drugs.

(My husband was one of them) From the statistics, more people die with low cholesterol than with high cholesterol. Your body actually needs some cholesterol. Statistics have proven this! [8][9]

The drug companies came up with a big scare in 1983 about cholesterol being too high. Could it be because they had come up with a drug that was supposed to lower cholesterol?

The drug companies conducted a poll that revealed they had the most problems convincing doctors that high cholesterol was dangerous to your health. But the drug companies put on such an advertising campaign that the public started requesting the cholesterol lowering "cure." Consumers were convinced by years of powerful, manipulative advertising.

The big wigs claimed cholesterol higher than 240 was dangerous. From where did this number originate? One-fourth of all adults have cholesterol above 240. That's a lot of people in need of treatment. And just think of the money treating twenty-five percent of the adult population would mean for them.

Apparently twenty-five percent wasn't enough of the population for the drug companies, so they changed the figures to below 200. That figure takes in just about everyone. According to the Douglass Report [10], cholesterol below 200 is actually dangerous. If yours is below 200, go to an *alternative* doctor immediately. Between 200 and 240 is normal cholesterol.

After all the advertising about lowering cholesterol to below 200, and people asking requesting the drugs, doctors started giving in. The newer doctors don't know any better; this is what they learn in medical school.

The difference of HDL and LDL is more important than the numbers themselves. If your cholesterol does need lowering, a natural statin, such as red yeast rice can lower it, although it doesn't cure a heart disease any more than the statin drugs.

On May 20, 2011 on the WXYZ TV channel, (Detroit area) the news reported "cooked tomatoes do as much good as any statin drugs."[11] This could include such yummy things as stewed tomatoes, as well as tomato paste and tomato juice. Tomato soup is best if homemade. This cure is cheap, delicious, and has no side effects!

Tomatoes contain high levels of lycopene, which fights free radicals (trouble makers) that can damage cells throughout your entire body. Harvard Medical School conducted a study of 50,000 men who ate lots of tomatoes had healthier prostates than men who did not.

Watermelon also contains lycopene, which isn't just for men—it fights all free radicals.

Recently, I was reading in one of our many Health Newsletters, "The Second Opinion," by Dr. Robert J. Rowen, MD, that you can't beat the beet. [12]

If you are one of fifty million Americans with hypertension, the simple beet is not only good to lower your blood pressure, it is also said to be effective for arthritis, colon cancer, chest pain, erectile dysfunction, and much more!

In a study done in London subjects were given beet juice to drink. Within one hour their blood pressure dropped considerably. Their blood pressure also stayed down for twenty-four hours. This sure "beets" the results from most drugs! In one of the studies triglycerides were reduced by forty percent and overall cholesterol dropped by thirty percent.

Beets are cheap and easy to grow. Their colorful leaves make a nice background as a border for flowers around the house. The beet is easily stored. They can be juiced, for those of you that have a juicer. Beets can be eaten raw or cooked. Borscht is a favorite of the Russians. The Polish, I believe, also use beets in a lot of their recipes. So, beets are certainly worth adding to your diet. They are great for your entire body.

One year my husband and I took a class from Mr. Agari, who once had one of his hands crushed by heavy machinery where he worked. The doctors wanted to amputate his hand, but he had heard of the wonder cures of many botanicals. He used what he already knew and continued to learn about plants, both for eating and applying. He held up both hands and asked if any of us could tell which hand had been crushed. No one could. He then took us on a field trip out behind the school to show us different plants and what their uses. Later he had "food" for us to try from the various plants. We learned certain plants that come out in different seasons have their own purpose. For instance dandelion, which comes out in the spring, is a good blood thinner—preparing us for warmer weather and increased activity. Sumac, which comes out later in the summer, makes a great drink that tastes like lemonade. (Use only the red sumac berries, the yellow variety is poisonous.) Oh, the wonders the good Lord provided for us humans!

A Personal Case History

In 2009, when my husband and I were in Florida for January, February, and March—our annual retreat from Michigan's cold winters—my husband was having some chest pains and an upset stomach in the middle of the night on a Tuesday. The combination of the two symptoms is not a good sign. We called 911, and not one but two ambulances and about a dozen people arrived in a very short time. The EMTs took my husband to Health Central Hospital, where the staff performed a cardiac catheterization, which revealed a blockage in some of his arteries.

The staff then sent him from there to what they called "The Big House," the Orlando Regional Medical Center—a hospital in downtown Orlando, Florida. The doctor there said my husband should have bypass surgery. He asked, "How much longer might I have?" The doctor answered, "It could be Thursday or it might be years." When my husband said he didn't want the bypass surgery, the doctor then exclaimed, "Then it's Thursday!" With that life threatening scare, my husband consented to having the surgery.

We wondered later if the doctor claimed it would be "Thursday" because he saw several thousands of dollars slipping away. While waiting for my husband in surgery, I was talking to a lady whose husband was also having bypass surgery. She said it was her husband's sixth bypass operation and that the doctors didn't give her much hope of his survival. (He did survive—at least he was alive right after the surgery. But who knows for how long after his release?)

My husband's quadruple bypass surgery was "needed" after we had been on the American Heart Associations recommended diet for several years. We ate low fat this, low fat that, the recommended margarine, and so on. After the surgery, my husband was sent to "rehab," which included using various exercise equipment and taking various classes. One of the classes was on diet. The instructor had product samples to show the "good foods" we should be consuming. Her samples looked like what used to be found in our cupboards and refrigerator! Another little-known fact is that margarine is actually made from a petroleum product. Petroleum may be great fuel for vehicles, but, our bodies do not need this kind of fuel.

One of the alternative health doctors in one of his newsletters said, "The more man messes with a food, the more you should leave it alone!" [13] This seems to include most of the foods recommended by the American Heart Association. More of man's messing with our foods.

The following is another anecdote about the side effects of the prescription medicines my husband was taking. He was told he needed to take a statin drug because of his previous bypass surgery. He started having some unusual reactions—dizziness, weakness, loss of appetite, fuzzy thinking, blood in the urine, and others. We decided we should read the literature that comes with prescriptions on possible side effects. The symptoms he was experiencing were all listed, and more. He stopped taking the prescriptions on March 3, 2011 and ten days later, the side effects continued. We were told later that he shouldn't stop a medicine all at once, that one should taper off slowly. Reason tells me this would just prolong the side effects. If a drug is causing serious side effects and perhaps killing you, why in the world would you continue to take any of it? This kind of logic mystifies me.

When we go to Florida for the winter, we live in a class "C" RV, with the bed over the cab. Usually my Husband puts his foot on the seat to the eating area below to get down. After the surgery, he was too weak to move over far enough and only had a couple of toes touching the seat. Suddenly he fell and hit his head very hard on the floor. He just missed a sharp corner of a TV tray. He must have passed out, because he does not remember falling. It took us over an hour to get him up on the couch though he had landed right next to it. He was too weak to get himself up, and I couldn't lift him. This was one of the drug's "on" times.

The following pictures show his black and blue forehead and eye, as well as a thumb and knee after the fall. He also had a sore hip and turned very yellow all over his body. The yellowing usually signals a problem with the liver.

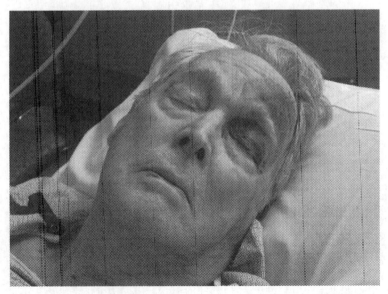

Black and blue forehead and eye from the fall demonstrating the side effect of "weakness" from statin drugs.

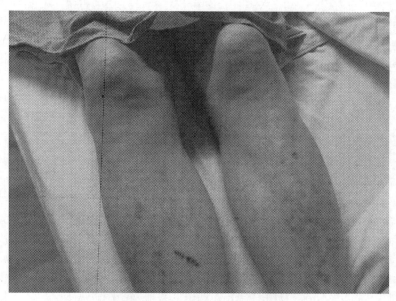

Black and blue knees from fall demonstrating the side effect of "weakness" from statin drugs.

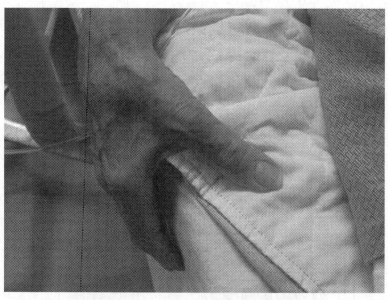

Black and blue hand from fall caused by side effect of "weakness" from statin drugs.

He was feeling a bit stronger in the morning after the fall (during one of the drug's "off" times) so we went to the emergency department at Health Central Hospital in Ocoee, Florida again, where he ended up seeing several specialists for his kidneys, heart, liver, and blood. He took many, many tests to find out what was causing his problems. Doctors took over forty x-rays, two MRI's, multiple CT scans, two ultrasounds, and blood tests several times a day. The blood platelets should be around 150, and they were down to only fifteen. The bilirubin (liver) count was twelve and it should have been about one or two.

One doctor did say he thought it was the result of the medicine my husband was taking, but Chuck (my husband) still had to go through all the testing to eliminate what or wasn't the cause of his problem. After all of these tests, it did end up that the cause of his problems *was* the Simvastatin he had been prescribed by a cardiologist.

As we were told, side effects can last for months, until the medications are totally gone from the person's system. Chuck was given several IV's daily to flush his system. This, flushing of the medication, certainly isn't in keeping with the idea of tapering off of a drug.

While he was undergoing all of these procedures we decided to incorporate some of the health information we had read about fairly recently. The three most important nutrients that we have found that the body needs are Vitamin C, calcium, and Vitamin D. Chuck ordered two orange juices for each of his meals. I put a package of Emergen-C, which contains 1000 mg of vitamin C each, in each of the juices. He was also taking several Ester-C pills (500 mg each). He further increased his vitamin C consumption with the chewable tablets with 500 mg each. In addition, he was taking six of the Barefoot Calcium Complete capsules (1,500 mg each) every day. These supplements were not taken with the approval of the medical personnel—they were not made aware we were doing it, and for good reason!

The Emergen-C packets, vitamin C pills and chewable tablets can be obtained at Walmart, Sam's Club, and Costco, among other stores. We get ours from Sam's Club, which has a better price than even Walmart.

Sam's Club used to carry the Mr. Barefoot Calcium Complete capsules, but have discontinued them. They were about $36 for a bottle of 240 capsules. We called the phone number on the bottle and now get them for close to the wholesale price ($19.95 each) by ordering a minimum of 6 bottles at a time. This is a great bargain for your health (and no side effects). These calcium capsules are premium grade from Okinawa, Japan, home to some of healthiest people on the planet! Thousands of this island's residents live to be over 100 years old. There are more centenarians in Okinawa than anywhere else in the world! In fact, at one time, most of the doctors left because of the lack of business. This was known as "The Japanese Exodus".

We used to think that one only needed to take vitamin C when you were coming down with a cold. But according to Dr. Levy, Dr. Pauling, scientist "Mr. Robert R. Barefoot", and other alternative doctors, you need vitamin C in every cell of your body, every day. They also tell you that you need calcium and vitamin D in every cell of your body. So, these very important vitamins and minerals need to be consumed every day for good health!

Both vitamin C and calcium have been proven to cure cancer as well as many other diseases. Don't leave home without them!

Along with several other vitamins, we take the most of the Coral Calcium Complete and vitamin C. We take six Coral Calcium Complete tablets and 6 Ester-C tablets per day—two of each in the morning, two of each at midday, and two of each in the evening. We also use a teaspoonful of Super C22, a packet of Emergen-C, one drop of iodine, and about ten drops of Reishi extract in a fruit drink (eight ounces) in the morning.

Reishi is a mushroom with over 150 known nutrients and antioxidant. It is great for the immune system, and boasts a whole lot of other beneficial health needs, like curing cancer. It is not cheap; East Earth Trade Winds is the least expensive brand we've located.

A one-ounce bottle is $20.95. We much prefer the liquid over the capsules because it's very easy to add to almost anything.

The address is:
East Earth Trade Winds
P.O. Box 493151
Redding, CA 96049
Phone 530-223-4849, Fax 530-223-0944

The 240-count Coral Calcium Complete is $19.95 per bottle when purchasing a minimum of six bottles. We purchase ours from:

NFI Consumer Products
4525 Campground Rd.
Fayetteville, NC 28414
Phone: toll free 800-432-9334 or 910-860-9740
Fax; 910-860-9742

This may start to sound expensive, but just try getting sick and you'll see what high costs really are!

Vitamin D is acquired by getting some sunshine. In spite of what we are being told about how bad sunshine is for you. Sunshine does not give you cancer, but some of the sun protection creams and lotions we are told we need to use can give you cancer! If you burn easily, stay in the shade and you will still get the needed vitamin D. Thirty minutes per day is all that is needed but, of course, more is even better. [14]

Were you aware that people that live closer to the equator (where they get lots of sun, rarely (if ever) get multiple sclerosis (MS)? The Lord did not make a big goof when He created the sun—He has never made a mistake and He never will!

You can also purchase vitamin D and eat foods that contain vitamin D. This is good any time, but especially beneficial when the sun is scarce.

We have read in the literature from several different doctor's newsletters and other materials that lecithin granules (about 1 tablespoon) will clean the arteries of plaque in as little as three weeks. If you continue to use it, it will keep them clean. Lecithin granules are also recommended by several of the alternative doctors. Lecithin promotes a healthy heart and improves circulation, in addition to helping brain and a liver function.

We put Lecithin granules on our cereal every day. We use yogurt, instead of milk, with our cereal, so the lecithin doesn't sink to the bottom. An airline stewardess told us how good yogurt is on cereal. We tried it and liked it with the yogurt. The lecithin granules have very little taste and are also good in oatmeal, on salads, in soup, and many other dishes. Lecithin is available in most health food stores. We like GNC's. Some of the other brands that we have tried have been powdery or tend to stick together and clump.

Fiber is very important, a good protection against heart disease. Put some ground flax seed into your daily diet. Flax seed has a nice nutty flavor. The whole flax seed needs to be ground for it to be beneficial to your health. We put some on our cereal in the morning along with the lecithin granules. It can also be used in a lot of different recipes.

Pre-ground flax seed can become rancid, so fresh ground is better. We use an Ultimate Chopper. (They used to be advertised a lot on TV.) We have had it for some years, but you could probably find it on the internet. This chopper is good for grinding small amounts.

If you want to try a pre-ground flax seed there is one carried by several grocery stores made by Hodgson Mill.

Another great machine for grinding larger items, such as wheat or other grains, making smoothies, shakes, juice (while retaining all the fiber), soups, and ice cream is the Vitamix blender. It's best for larger quantities. We use ours almost every day!

Vitamix
8615 Usher Road
Cleveland, Ohio 44138-2199
Phone: 800-848-2649 440-235-4840

Our favorite books on having good health and what we strongly recommend everyone getting are:

"The One Minute Cure", by Madison Cavanaugh Think Outside the Book Publishing.

Curing the Incurable: Vitamin C, Infectious Diseases, and Toxins, by Thomas E. Levy, MD, JD (with over 1,200 scientific references). 1-866-790-2107 code CTIR $19.95 (as of this writing).

The Disease Conspiracy: The FDA Suppression of Cures, by Robert R. Barefoot. 1-800-432-9334

The Calcium Factor: The Scientific Secret of Health and Youth, by Robert R. Barefoot and Carl J. Reich, MD. This is also obtained through the phone number above.

Why We Get Fat and What to Do About It, by Gary Taubes. $24.95 in most book stores. It is far more about having a very good heart and good health than just losing weight. This is another must-have book!

Following are several pages of the reports that my husband received to take back to our doctor in Michigan. Some of it will probably not be very understandable to many of us, but any doctor will understand these reports. Our doctor in Michigan and the last one Chuck saw in Florida said he came "close to checking out" and that Chuck was "lucky to still be here." This was not because of anything we had done or didn't do, but because of what one of the "wonder drugs" prescribed by a cardiologist had done to him.

We believe he *is* lucky to be here because of the large doses of vitamin C and calcium that he was taking, along with the IV's to flush his system, while he was in the hospital. We also think the vitamin C and calcium was why the doctors in Florida said he was making "a very good recovery" and even "a remarkable recovery."

Even if you do not understand what is on the following pages, it is proof that he was in the hospital and underwent a lot of tests. It is not something we made up to write about!

Patient Name: EVERY,CHARLES   All Sections-Page 1
Med Rec #:   487530   Adm: 03/15/11
Dis Date: 03/22/11
Phys-Service: NANDLALL,BANEY P - PROGESSIVE CARE
Acct #:   A1107400220
****

HEMATOLOGY

Date:	03/22	03/21	03/20	03/19	03/18	Reference Range	
Time:	0456	0408	0521	0415	1115		
New Work:	*	PREV RPT	PREV RPT	PREV RPT	PREV RPT		
WBC	7.6	7.3	6.3	6.3	6.4	3.6-9.8	{K/mm3}
Corr WBC				6.2	6.3	3.6-9.8	{K/mm3}
RBC	3.20 L	3.10 L	3.10 L	3.20 L	3.16 L	4.14-5.70	{m/mm3}
Hgb	10.2 L	10.1 L	10.0 L	10.3 L	10.3 L	13.5-18.0	{gm/dL}
Hct	32.5 L	31.1 L	31.0 L	31.1 L	30.6 L	38.0-48.0	{%}
MCV	102 H	100 H	100 H	97 H	97 H	81.6-94.8	{fL}
MCH	31.9	32.6	32.3	32.2	32.6	27.5-32.8	{pg}
MCHC	31.4 L	32.5 L	32.3 L	33.1	33.7	33.1-35.2	{%}
RDW	17.9 H	17.6 H	17.1 H	16.7 H	16.6 H	11.4-15.7	{%}
Platelet	89 L	85 L	71 L	65 L	60 L	150-450	{K/mm3}
MPV	10.0	10.8 H	10.0	10.7 H	10.7 H	6.9-10.5	{fL}
Segs				70	55	50-70	{%}
Bands				1	10	0-15	{%}
Lymphs				13	9	0-30	{%}
Mono				15 H	20 H	1-6	{%}
Eos				1	3	0-3	{%}
Var Lym				3	3	0-15	{%}
NRBC				1 H	1 H	0-0	{ /100WB
RBC Morph				#	Normal		
Plt Est				#	#		

HEMATOLOGY

Date:	03/17	03/16	03/15			Reference Range	
Time:	0440	0909	1420				
New Work:	PREV RPT	PREV RPT	PREV RPT				
WBC	4.9	6.5	11.6 H			3.6-9.8	{K/mm3}
RBC	3.13 L	3.29 L	3.89 L			4.14-5.70	{m/mm3}
Hgb	10.1 L	10.6 L	12.9 L			13.5-18.0	{gm/dL}
Hct	30.9 L	32.2 L	38.1			38.0-48.0	{%}
MCV	99 H	98 H	98 H			81.6-94.8	{fL}
MCH	32.3	32.2	33.2 H			27.5-32.8	{pg}
MCHC	32.7 L	32.9 L	33.9			33.1-35.2	{%}
RDW	16.7 H	16.5 H	16.7 H			11.4-15.7	{%}
Platelet	52 L	52 L	61 L			150-450	{K/mm3}
MPV	10.7 H	10.0	10.3			6.9-10.5	{fL}
Neutro		66.6	77.9 H			44.2-73.2	{%}

Continued next page

M.R.Sherman,MD-LAB/T.Wentzell,MD-R.T.   EVERY,CHARLES
Health Central Laboratory   487530
Ocoee, FL 34761
** DO NOT DISCARD **   (M-02/24/30)
Discharge Cumulative Trend Report   Dr. NANDLALL,BANEY P

Patient Name:	EVERY,CHARLES	All Sections-Page 2
Med Rec #:	487530	Adm: 03/15/11
Dis Date	03/22/11	
Phys-Service:	NANDLALL,BANEY P - PROGESSIVE CARE	
Acct #:	A1107400220	

****

~~~~~~

HEMATOLOGY (Cont)

Date:	03/17	03/16	03/15			Reference Range
Time:	0440	0909	1420			
New Work:	PREV RPT	PREV RPT	PREV RPT			
IG			0.4			0.0-2.0 (%)
Lymph		5.9 L	5.3 L			15.2-42.7 (%)
Monos		25.6 H	16.0 H			4.3-11.6 (%)
Eos		0.5	0.1 L			0.2-6.8 (%)
Baso		0.8	0.3			0.1-1.8 (%)

- - - - - - - - - - - - - - - Specific Comments - - - - - - - - - - - - - -
03/19/11 0415|CBC W/DIFF-RBC Morph: 1+ Anisocytosis
03/19/11 0415|CBC W/DIFF-Plt Est: Markedly Decreased
03/18/11 1115|CBC W/DIFF-Plt Est: Markedly Decreased
~~~~~~

COAGULATION

Date:	03/17	03/17	03/15			Reference Range
Time:	1015	0440	1420			
New Work:	PREV RPT	PREV RPT	PREV RPT			
Protime		11.4	11.1			9.2-12.5 (secs)
INR		1.07	1.04			Therap 2.0-3.0
PTT		35.2 H	36.2 H			24.4-34.0 (secs)
Fibrinogen		559.8 H				200-500 (mg/dl)
D-Dimer	1.50 H					0.19-0.6 (mg/L)

CHEMISTRY

Date:	03/22	03/21	03/20	03/19	03/18	Reference Range
Time:	0456	0408	0521	0415	1115	
New Work:	PREV RPT	PREV RPT	PREV RPT	PREV RPT	PREV RPT	
Glucose	84	88	86			71-113 (mg/dl)
BUN	15	14	15			7-19 (mg/dl)
Creatinine	1.1	1.1	1.2			0.4-1.4 (mg/dl)
Sodium	134 L	136	136			135-147 (mEq/L)
Potassium	3.8	4.0	4.1			3.6-5.2 (mEq/L)

Continued next page

M.R.Sherman,MD-LAB/T.Wentzell,MD-R.T.	EVERY,CHARLES
Health Central Laboratory	487530
Ocoee, FL 34761	
** DO NOT DISCARD **	(M-02/24/30)
Discharge Cumulative Trend Report	Dr. NANDLALL,BANEY P

Patient Name: EVERY,CHARLES   All Sections-Page 3
Med Rec #:   487530   Adm: 03/15/11
Dis Date: 03/22/11
Phys-Service: NANDLALL,BANEY P - PROGESSIVE CARE
Acct #:   A1107400220
****

CHEMISTRY (Cont)

Date:	03/22	03/21	03/20	03/19	03/18	Reference Range
Time:	0456	0408	0521	0415	1115	
New Work:	PREV RPT	PREV RPT	PREV RPT	PREV RPT	PREV RPT	
Chloride	100	102	102			98-110 (mEq/L)
CO2	26.9	26.3	25.8			20.3-30.3 (mmol/L)
Calcium	8.6	8.1	8.2			8.0-10.0 (mg/dl)
Bilirubin, T	3.6 H	4.3 HP	4.8 HP	7.0 HP		0.0-1.3 (mg/dl)
Bilirubin, D				5.70 HP		0.0-0.2 (mg/dl)
Protein,Total	6.3 L	6.1 L	5.9 L	5.9 L		6.4-8.2 (gm/dl)
Albumin	2.6 L	2.6 L	2.4 L	2.5 L		3.1-4.7 (gm/dl)
Ammonia					14	11-32 (umol/L)
ENZYMES						
Alk Phos	427 H	430 H	388 H	372 H		31-135 (IU/L)
AST (SGOT)	64 H	64 H	64 H	65 H		1-37 (IU/L)
ALT (SGPT)	106 H	103 H	98 H	100 H		20-56 (IU/L)

CHEMISTRY

Date:	03/18	03/18	03/17	03/17	03/16	Reference Range
Time:	1115	0445	0440	0440	0510	
New Work:	PREV RPT	PREV RPT	PREV RPT	PREV RPT	PREV RPT	
Glucose	114 H	105	100			71-113 (mg/dl)
BUN	14	14	20 H			7-19 (mg/dl)
Creatinine	1.0	1.1	1.2			0.4-1.4 (mg/dl)
Sodium	133 L	136	135			135-147 (mEq/L)
Potassium	3.9	3.8	3.7			3.6-5.2 (mEq/L)
Chloride	102	103	102			98-110 (mEq/L)
CO2	24.0	23.6	25.4			20.3-30.3 (mmol/L)
Calcium	7.9 L	7.9 L	8.2			8.0-10.0 (mg/dl)
Bilirubin, T	9.5 HP		14.4 HP		14.0 HP	0.0-1.3 (mg/dl)
Bilirubin, D					12.00 HP	0.0-0.2 (mg/dl)
Protein,Total	5.5 L		5.4 L		5.8 L	6.4-8.2 (gm/dl)
Albumin	2.4 L		2.4 L		2.5 L	3.1-4.7 (gm/dl)
ENZYMES						
Alk Phos	365 H		278 H		225 H	31-135 (IU/L)
AST (SGOT)	83 H		106 H		125 H	1-37 (IU/L)
ALT (SGPT)	109 H		106 H		112 H	20-56 (IU/L)
Amylase				131 H		21-103 (IU/L)
Lipase				1071 H		105 - 265 (U/L)

Continued next page

M.R.Sherman,MD-LAB/T.Wentzell,MD-R.T.   EVERY,CHARLES
Health Central Laboratory   487530
Ocoee, FL 34761
** DO NOT DISCARD **   (M-02/24/30)
Discharge Cumulative Trend Report   Dr. NANDLALL,BANEY P

Patient Name: EVERY,CHARLES   All Sections-Page 4
Med Rec #:   487530   Adm: 03/15/11
Dis Date   03/22/11
Phys-Service: NANDLALL,BANEY P - PROGESSIVE CARE
Acct #:   A1107400220

****

~~~~~~

CHEMISTRY (Cont)

Date:	03/16	03/15				Reference Range
Time:	0510	1420				
New Work:	PREV RPT	PREV RPT				

Glucose		118 H				71-113	(mg/dl)
BUN		27 H				7-19	(mg/dl)
Creatinine		1.7 H				0.4-1.4	(mg/dl)
Sodium		134 L				135-147	(mEq/L)
Potassium		3.8				3.6-5.2	(mEq/L)
Chloride		98				98-110	(mEq/L)
CO2		24.4				20.3-30.3	(mmol/L)
Calcium		9.0				8.0-10.0	(mg/dl)
Bilirubin, T		15.6 H				0.0-1.3	(mg/dl)
Protein,Total		6.8				6.4-8.2	(gm/dl)
Albumin		3.0 L				3.1-4.7	(gm/dl)
ENZYMES							
Alk Phos		225 H				31-135	(IU/L)
AST (SGOT)		128 H				1-37	(IU/L)
ALT (SGPT)		107 H				20-56	(IU/L)
LDH Total	287 H					112-204	(IU/L)
Lipase		501 H				105 - 265	(U/L)

~~~~~~

WB Glucose

Date:	03/18					Reference Range
Time:	1639					
New Work:	PREV RPT					

WB Glucose	110					71-113	(mg/dl)

Patient Name: EVERY,CHARLES   All Sections-Page 5
Med Rec #:   487530   Adm: 03/15/11
Dis Date   03/22/11
Phys-Service: NANDLALL,BANEY P - PROGESSIVE CARE
Acct #:   A1107400220
****

GFR

Date:	03/22	03/21	03/20	03/18	03/18	Reference Range	
Time:	0456	0408	0521	1115	0445		
New Work:	PREV RPT	PREV RPT	PREV RPT	PREV RPT	PREV RPT		
Creatinine	1.1	1.1	1.2	1.0	1.1	0.4~1.4	(mg/dL)
GFR	>60	>60	>60	>60	>60	>60	(mL/min/

GFR

Date:	03/17	03/15				Reference Range	
Time:	0440	1420					
New Work:	PREV RPT	PREV RPT					
Creatinine	1.2	1.7 H				0.4~1.4	(mg/dL)
GFR	>60	41 L				>60	(mL/min/

SPECIAL CHEMISTRY

Date:	03/17	03/17				Reference Range	
Time:	0440	0440					
New Work:	PREV RPT	PREV RPT					
Iron	58					40~156	(ug/dl)
TIBC	421					250~400	(ug/ml)
Ferritin		519 H				F 10~130 M 26~246	

In: 03/17/11 0547   --------   Spec: Blood
Out: 03/17/11 0927 | PSA | Techs: VPMB TJFB
Coll Time: 03/17/11 0440   --------
Order Phys: ABREU,ELPIDIO A   [A1107400220/2916503]

Result Name	Result	Reference Range
PSA(ng/ml):	1.3	<4.0

Patient Name: EVERY,CHARLES   All Sections-Page 6
Med Rec #:   487530   Adm: 03/15/11
Dis Date   03/22/11
Phys-Service: NANDLALL,BANEY P - PROGESSIVE CARE
Acct #:   A1107400220
****

In: 03/16/11 1006   --------   Spec: Blood
Out: 03/16/11 1212 | PSA | Techs: VCAK1 TJFB
Coll Time: 03/16/11 0510   --------
Order Phys: NANDLALL,BANEY P   {A1107400220/2916270}

Result Name   Result   Reference Range

PSA(ng/ml):   1.1   <4.0

In: 03/15/11 1437   ----------------------------   Spec: Blood
Out: 03/15/11 1636 | TSH-3RD GENERATION | Techs: V-11922 TNR
Coll Time: 03/15/11 1420   ----------------------------
Order Phys: HOFF,LISA A   {A1107400220/2915381}
                           *STAT*STAT*STAT*
Result Name   Result   Reference Range

TSH, 3rd Generation(uIU/mL): 10.900 H   0.47-4.68

M.R.Sherman,MD-LAB/T.Wentzell,MD-R.T.   EVERY,CHARLES
Health Central Laboratory   487530
Ocoee, FL 34761
** DO NOT DISCARD **   {M-02/24/30}
Discharge Cumulative Trend Report   Dr. NANDLALL,BANEY P

Patient:EVERY, CHARLES   MRN:487530   Encounter:1107400220   Page 6 of 21

Patient Name: EVERY,CHARLES   All Sections-Page 7
Med Rec #:   487530   Adm: 03/15/11
Dis Date   03/22/11
Phys-Service: NANDLALL,BANEY P - PROGESSIVE CARE
Acct #:   A1107400220
****

CARDIAC MARKERS

Date:	03/21	03/17	03/16	03/15	03/15		
Time:	0408	0440	0510	2210	1420	Reference Range	
New Work:	PREV RPT	PREV RPT	PREV RPT	PREV RPT	PREV RPT		
CPK Total	66	532 H	821 H	1011 HP	1305 HP	0-218	(IU/L)
CK-MB	n/a	0.6	<0.5	<0.5	0.9	0.0-3.6	(ng/ml)
CK-MB Index	Not cal^	0.1	#	#	0.1	0.0-1.5	(%)
Troponin I	<0.04	<0.04	0.06	<0.04	0.05	0.00-0.07 ng/ml	

~ ~ ~ ~ ~ ~ ~ ~ ~ ~ ~ ~ ~ ~ Specific Comments ~ ~ ~ ~ ~ ~ ~ ~ ~ ~ ~ ~ ~ ~ ~
03/16/11 0510|CPK TOTAL-CK-MB Index: Not calc'd
03/15/11 2210|CPK TOTAL-CK-MB Index: Not calc'd
****

In: 03/15/11 1437   --------   Spec: Blood
Out: 03/15/11 1503 | BNP | Techs: V-11922 TNR
Coll Time: 03/15/11 1420   --------
Order Phys: HOFF,LISA A   {A1107400220/2915380}
                                * STAT*STAT*STAT*
Result Name   Result   Reference Range

Brain Natriuretic Pe(pg/mL):   307 H   0-100

****

M.R.Sherman,MD-LAB/T.Wentzell,MD-R.T.   EVERY,CHARLES
Health Central Laboratory   487530
Ocoee, FL 34761
** DO NOT DISCARD **   {M-02/24/30}
Discharge Cumulative Trend Report   Dr. NANDLALL,BANEY P

Patient:EVERY, CHARLES   MRN:487530   Encounter:1107400220   Page 7 of 21

Patient Name: EVERY,CHARLES   All Sections-Page 8
Med Rec #:   487530   Adm: 03/15/11
Dis Date   03/22/11
Phys-Service: NANDLALL,BANEY P - PROGESSIVE CARE
Acct #:   A1107400220
****

                              OSMOLALITY

Date: | 03/16 | | | | |
Time: | 1019 | | | | | Reference Range
New Work: |PREV RPT| | | | |

Osmol, Urine | 621 | | | | | 50-1400   (mOsm/kg

Patient Name: EVERY,CHARLES   URINALYSIS-Page 9
Med Rec #:   487530   Adm: 03/15/11
Dis Date   03/22/11
Phys-Service: NANDLALL,BANEY P - PROGESSIVE CARE
Acct #:   A1107400220
****

>> CULTURE, URINE <<
Source: Urine MSCC

Coll. Time: 03/15/11 1605   In at: 03/15/11 1650   Acct #: A1107400220
Order Phys: MASCOE,MAURICE W   Techs : V-11922
- -
Out at: 03/17/11 1040   Final {2915436}   Techs: THP*

CULTURE
No growth in 36-48 hours

~~~~~~

In: 03/15/11 1607   ~~~~~~~~~~~~~~~~~~~~   Spec: Urine MSCC
Out: 03/15/11 1650 | URINALYSIS SCREEN | Techs: V-11922 TCXV*
Coll Time: 03/15/11 1605 ~~~~~~~~~~~~~~~~~~~~
Order Phys: HOFF,LISA A   {A1107400220/2915436}

                          *STAT*STAT*STAT*
Result Name   Result

Color: Amber
Appearance: Clear
Glucose(mg/dl):   100 mg/dL
Ketones(mg/dl):   Trace
Blood: Negative
Protein(mg/dl):   30 mg/dL
Nitrite: Positive
Bile: Large
Spec Gravity: 1.025
pH: 5.5
Urobilinogen(EU/dl):   1.0 E.U./dL
Leukocytes: Trace
WBCs(/HPF):   3-5
RBCs(/HPF):   0-2
Bacteria: 1+
Epithelial Cell(/LPF):   1-4
Casts(/LPF):   0-2 Hyaline, 1-2 Granular
Culture in Progress: Yes

~~~~~~

M.R.Sherman,MD-LAB/T.Wentzell,MD-R.T.   EVERY,CHARLES
Health Central Laboratory   487530
Ocoee, FL 34761
** DO NOT DISCARD **   {M-02/24/30}
Discharge Cumulative Trend Report   Dr. NANDLALL,BANEY P

Patient Name: EVERY,CHARLES   REFERENCE LAB-Page 10
Med Rec #:   487530   Adm: 03/15/11
Dis Date   03/22/11
Phys-Service: NANDLALL,BANEY P - PROGESSIVE CARE
Acct #:   A1107400220
****

In: 03/21/11 1308   --------------------------------   Spec: Blood
Out: To follow | ALPHA-1-ANTITRYPSIN (8161) | Techs: VAMK
Coll Time: 03/21/11 0408--------------------------------
Order Phys: MEJIA,LUIS E   [A1107400220/2921533]

Result Name   Result   Reference Range

Reviewed by: To follow

                 Referred to: Mayo Reference Services
                              150 Third Street SW
                              Rochester, MN 55902

In: 03/21/11 1308   --------------------------------   Spec: Blood
Out: To follow | MITOCHONDRIAL AB, M2 (800086) | Techs: VAMK
Coll Time: 03/21/11 0408--------------------------------
Order Phys: MEJIA,LUIS E   [A1107400220/2921533]

Result Name   Result   Reference Range

Reviewed by: To follow

                 Referred to: Mayo Reference Services
                              150 Third Street SW
                              Rochester, MN 55902

In: 03/21/11 1308   --------------------------------   Spec: Blood
Out: To follow | CERULOPLASMIN (800104) | Techs: VAMK
Coll Time: 03/21/11 0408--------------------------------
Order Phys: MEJIA,LUIS E   [A1107400220/2921533]

Result Name   Result   Reference Range

Reviewed by: To follow

                 Referred to: Mayo Reference Services
                              150 Third Street SW
                              Rochester, MN 55902

M.R.Sherman,MD-LAB/T.Wentzell,MD-R.T.   EVERY,CHARLES
Health Central Laboratory   487530
Ocoee, FL 34761
** DO NOT DISCARD **   [M-02/24/30]
Discharge Cumulative Trend Report   Dr. NANDLALL,BANEY P

Patient Name: EVERY,CHARLES   REFERENCE LAB-Page 11
Med Rec #:   487530   Adm: 03/15/11
Dis Date   03/22/11
Phys-Service: NANDLALL,BANEY P - PROGESSIVE CARE
Acct #:   A1107400220
****

In: 03/17/11 0547   -------------------------------   Spec: Blood
Out: 03/21/11 1032 | ANTI-SMOOTH MUSCLE AB (800246) | Techs: VPMB TCLB
Coll Time: 03/17/11 0440-----------------------------------
Order Phys: NANDLALL,BANEY P   [A1107400220/2917075]

Result Name   Result   Reference Range

ANTI-SMOOTH MUSCL AB(Titer): SEE COMMENTS   NEGATIVE
                              03/21/2011 08/31 AM

Mayo:

                                          HI   Expected
Test   Result   LO Units   Values

Anti-Smooth Muscle Ab   Negative   Negative

   Test Performed by:
   Mayo Clinic Jacksonville Clinical Lab
   4500 San Pablo Rd, Jacksonville, FL 32224
   Laboratory Director: Arthur D. Jones, Jr. M.D.

Reviewed by: Carrie L Barron,

            Referred to: Mayo Reference Services
                         150 Third Street SW
                         Rochester, MN 55902

In: 03/17/11 0547   -------------------------------   Spec: Blood
Out: 03/18/11 0742 | AFP TUMOR MARKER (800002) | Techs: VPMB TCLB
Coll Time: 03/17/11 0440-----------------------------------
Order Phys: NANDLALL,BANEY P   [A1107400220/2917076]

Result Name   Result   Reference Range

AFP Tumor Marker(ng/mL):   SEE COMMENTS   <6.0
                              03/18/2011 02/26 AM

Mayo:

                                          HI   Expected
Test   Result   LO Units   Values

Alpha-Fetoprotein, Tumor Marker, S   1.2   ng/mL <6.0

                   {Continued on next page}
M.R.Sherman,MD-LAB/T.Wentzell,MD-R.T.   EVERY,CHARLES
Health Central Laboratory   487530
Ocoee, FL 34761
** DO NOT DISCARD **   {M-02/24/30)
Discharge Cumulative Trend Report   Dr. NANDLALL,BANEY P

Patient Name: EVERY,CHARLES   REFERENCE LAB-Page 12
Med Rec #:   487530   Adm: 03/15/11
Dis Date   03/22/11
Phys-Service: NANDLALL,BANEY P - PROGESSIVE CARE
Acct #:   A1107400220
****
In: 03/17/11 0547   --------------------------   Spec: Blood
Out: 03/18/11 0742 | AFP TUMOR MARKER (800002) | Techs: VPMB TCLB
Coll Time: 03/17/11 0440---------------------------------
Order Phys: NANDLALL,BANEY P   {A1107400220/2917076}

Result Name   Result   Reference Range

                     (Continued from previous page)
     The testing method is an immunoenzymatic assay manufactured
     by Beckman Coulter Inc. and performed on the Unicel DXI
     800.

     Values obtained with different assay methods or kits may
     be different and cannot be used interchangeably.

     Test results cannot be interpreted as absolute evidence for
     the presence or absence of malignant disease.

     Alpha-fetoprotein values are not interpretable in pregnant
     females for the investigation of malignant disease.

     Test Performed by:
     Mayo Clinic Jacksonville Clinical Lab
     4500 San Pablo Rd, Jacksonville, FL 32224
     Laboratory Director: Arthur D. Jones, Jr. M.D.

Reviewed by: Carrie L Barron,

            Referred to: Mayo Reference Services
                         150 Third Street SW
                         Rochester, MN 55902

M.R.Sherman,MD-LAB/T.Wentzell,MD-R.T.   EVERY,CHARLES
Health Central Laboratory   487530
Ocoee, FL 34761
** DO NOT DISCARD **   (M-02/24/30)
Discharge Cumulative Trend Report   Dr. NANDLALL,BANEY P

Patient Name: EVERY,CHARLES   REFERENCE LAB-Page 13
Med Rec #:   487530   Adm: 03/15/11
Dis Date   03/22/11
Phys-Service: NANDLALL,BANEY P - PROGRESSIVE CARE
Acct #:   A1107400220
****

In: 03/16/11 1138   -------------------------------   Spec: Bone Marrow
Out: 03/17/11 0940 | FLOW CYTOMETRY-LEUKEMIA PANEL | Techs: VDHW TCLB
Coll Time: 03/16/11 1040-----------------------------
Order Phys: NANDLALL,BANEY P   [A1107400220/2916301]

Result Name   Result   Reference Range

Flow Cytometry/Leukemia: See Ameripath Report   (Ref Lab report to chart)

In: 03/16/11 1430   ---------------------------------   Spec: Urine MSCC
Out: 03/22/11 0948 | IMMUNOFIXATION, URINE (8823) | Techs: VPCU TCLB
Coll Time: 03/16/11 1019------------------------------
Order Phys: ABREU,ELPIDIO A   [A1107400220/2916536]

Result Name   Result   Reference Range

Immunofixation, Urine: SEE COMMENTS   No Monoclonal Protein Detected
                           03/21/2011 12:59 PM

Mayo:

Test	Result	HI LO	Units	Expected Values
Monoclonal Protein Study, U				
Total Protein			mg/24 h	<102
Not a 24 hour collection; normals do not apply				
Collection Duration	Random		h	
Concentration	43		mg/dL	
Albumin	21		%	
Alpha 1-Globulin	16		%	
Alpha 2-Globulin	28		%	
Beta-Globulin	22		%	
Gamma-Globulin	12		%	
A/G Ratio	0.27			
Impression	See Ref Lab Comment			
All fractions present, no apparent M-spike.				
See Immunofixation				
Immunofixation, U				
No monoclonal protein detected.				

    Test Performed by:
    Mayo Clinic Dpt of Lab Med and Pathology

                        (Continued on next page)
M.R.Sherman,MD-LAB/T.Wentzell,MD-R.T.   EVERY,CHARLES
Health Central Laboratory   487530
Ocoee, FL 34761
** DO NOT DISCARD **   (M-02/24/30)
Discharge Cumulative Trend Report   Dr. NANDLALL,BANEY P

Patient Name: EVERY,CHARLES   REFERENCE LAB-Page 14
Med Rec #:   487530   Adm: 03/15/11
Dis Date   03/22/11
Phys-Service: NANDLALL,BANEY P - PROGESSIVE CARE
Acct #:   A1107400220
****

In: 03/16/11 1430   ----------------------------------   Spec: Urine MSCC
Out: 03/22/11 0948 | IMMUNOFIXATION, URINE (8823) | Techs: VPCU TCLB
Coll Time: 03/16/11 1019---------------------------------------
Order Phys: ABREU,ELPIDIO A   [A1107400220/2916536]

Result Name   Result   Reference Range

                    [Continued from previous page]
       200 first Street SW, Rochester, MN 55905
       Laboratory Director: Franklin R. Cockerill, III, M.D.

Reviewed by: Carrie L Barron,

                Referred to: Mayo Reference Services
                            150 Third Street SW
                            Rochester, MN 55902

In: 03/16/11 1006   ----------------------------------   Spec: Blood
Out: 03/21/11 1045 | MONOCLONAL PROTEIN STUDY, S 81756 | Techs: VCAK1 TCLB
Coll Time: 03/16/11 0510-------------------------------------
Order Phys: NANDLALL,BANEY P   [A1107400220/2916273]

Result Name   Result   Reference Range

Mayo:

Test	Result	HI LO	Units	Expected Values
Monoclonal Protein Study, S				
Total Protein	5.5	1	g/dL	6.3-7.9
Albumin	2.7	1	g/dL	3.4-4.7
Alpha-1 Globulin	0.3		g/dL	0.1-0.3
Alpha-2 Globulin	0.8		g/dL	0.6-1.0
Beta-Globulin	0.9		g/dL	0.7-1.2
Gamma-Globulin	0.8		g/dL	0.6-1.6
A/G Ratio	0.93			
Impression	See Ref Lab Comment			

     No apparent monoclonal protein on serum electrophoresis.
     See Immunofixation
   Immunofixation
     No monoclonal protein detected.

                    [Continued on next page]
M.R.Sherman,MD-LAB/T.Wentzell,MD-R.T.   EVERY,CHARLES
Health Central Laboratory   487530
Ocoee, FL 34761
** DO NOT DISCARD **   [M-02/24/30]
Discharge Cumulative Trend Report   Dr. NANDLALL,BANEY P

Patient Name: EVERY,CHARLES   REFERENCE LAB-Page 15
Med Rec #:   487530   Adm: 03/15/11
Dis Date   03/22/11
Phys-Service: NANDLALL,BANEY P - PROGRESSIVE CARE
Acct #:   A1107400220
****
In: 03/16/11 1006 -----------------------------------   Spec: Blood
Out: 03/21/11 1045 | MONOCLONAL PROTEIN STUDY, S 81756 | Techs: VCAK1 TCLB
Coll Time: 03/16/11 0510--------------------------------------
Order Phys: NANDLALL,BANEY P   [A1107400220/2916273]

Result Name   Result   Reference Range

                        (Continued from previous page)

     Test Performed by:
     Mayo Clinic Dpt of Lab Med and Pathology
     200 First Street SW, Rochester, MN 55905
     Laboratory Director: Franklin R. Cockerill, III, M.D.

Reviewed by: Carrie L Barron,
Alpha 1(gm/dL):   SEE COMMENTS   0.1-0.3
                             03/18/2011 04/02 PM

               Referred to: Mayo Reference Services
                            150 Third Street SW
                            Rochester, MN 55902

~~~~~~

M.R.Sherman,MD-LAB/T.Wentzell,MD-R.T.   EVERY,CHARLES
Health Central Laboratory   487530
Ocoee, FL 34761
** DO NOT DISCARD **   (M-02/24/30)
Discharge Cumulative Trend Report   Dr. NANDLALL,BANEY P

Patient Name: EVERY,CHARLES   MICROBIOLOGY-Page 16
Med Rec #:   487530   Adm: 03/15/11
Dis Date   03/22/11
Phys-Service: NANDLALL,BANEY P - PROGRESSIVE CARE
Acct #:   A1107400220
****

>> CULTURE, BLOOD <<
Source: Blood
Coll. Time: 03/17/11 0455   In at: 03/17/11 0556   Acct #: A1107400220
Order Phys: NANDLALL,BANEY P   Techs : VPMB
- -
Out at: 03/22/11 1002   Final [2917077]   Techs: THP*

ACCN COMMENT: -right ac
BLOOD CULTURE
No growth in 5 days

~~~~~~

>> CULTURE, BLOOD <<
Source: Blood
Coll. Time: 03/17/11 0440   In at: 03/17/11 0547   Acct #: A1107400220
Order Phys: NANDLALL,BANEY P   Techs : VPMB
- -
Out at: 03/22/11 1011   Final [2917076]   Techs: THP*

BLOOD CULTURE
No growth in 5 days

~~~~~~

M.R.Sherman,MD-LAB/T.Wentzell,MD-R.T.   EVERY,CHARLES
Health Central Laboratory   487530
Ocoee, FL 34761
** DO NOT DISCARD **   (M-02/24/30)
Discharge Cumulative Trend Report   Dr. NANDLALL,BANEY P

Patient Name: EVERY,CHARLES   MICROBIOLOGY-Page 16
Med Rec #:   487530   Adm: 03/15/11
Dis Date   03/22/11
Phys-Service: NANDLALL,BANEY P - PROGESSIVE CARE
Acct #:   A1107400220
****
                      >> CULTURE, BLOOD <<
                        Source: Blood
Coll. Time: 03/17/11 0455   In at: 03/17/11 0556   Acct #: A1107400220
Order Phys: NANDLALL,BANEY P   Techs: VPMB
- -
Out at: 03/22/11 1002   Final {2917077}   Techs: THP*

ACCN COMMENT: -right ac
BLOOD CULTURE
No growth in 5 days

~~~~~~

                      >> CULTURE, BLOOD <<
                        Source: Blood
Coll. Time: 03/17/11 0440   In at: 03/17/11 0547   Acct #: A1107400220
Order Phys: NANDLALL,BANEY P   Techs : VPMB
- -
Out at: 03/22/11 1011   Final {2917676}   Techs: THP*

BLOOD CULTURE
No growth in 5 days

~~~~~~

M.R.Sherman,MD-LAB/T.Wentzell,MD-R.T.   EVERY,CHARLES
Health Central Laboratory   487530
Ocoee, FL 34761
** DO NOT DISCARD **   {M-02/24/30)
Discharge Cumulative Trend Report   Dr. NANDLALL,BANEY P

Patient Name: EVERY,CHARLES   Page 17
Med Rec #:   487530   Adm: 03/15/11
Dis Date   03/22/11
Phys-Service: NANDLALL,BANEY P - PROGESSIVE CARE
Acct #:   A1107400220
****

Accession Number	Test Name	Spec Type	Collection Date & Time	Status
2921533	ALPHA-1-ANTITRYPSIN (8161)	Blood	03/21/11 0408	Transmit
2921533	MITOCHONDRIAL AB, M2 (80008)	Blood	03/21/11 0408	Transmit
2921533	CERULOPLASMIN (800104)	Blood	03/21/11 0408	Transmit

End of Report
****

M.R.Sherman,MD-LAB/T.Wentzell,MD-R.T.   EVERY,CHARLES
Health Central Laboratory   487530
Ocoee, FL 34761
** DO NOT DISCARD **   (M-02/24/30)
Discharge Cum Incomplete Work Listing   Dr. NANDLALL,BANEY P

Patient Name: EVERY,CHARLES   Notification-Page 18
Med Rec #:   487530   Adm: 03/15/11
Dis Date   03/22/11
Phys-Service: NANDLALL,BANEY P - PROGRESSIVE CARE
Acct #:   A1107400220
****

              LABORATORY CANCELLED AND SPECIMEN REJECTED TESTS

                    ****SPECIMEN REJECTED****
Accn: 2915379   Acct: A1107400220
Spec: Urine MSCC   Collected: 03/15/11 1510
Priority: *STAT*   Ord Phys: HOFF,LISA A

        Test Name: URINALYSIS SCREEN

        Rejected: 03/15/11 1529   Rejected by: IBS
        Rejection Reason: RN MISLABELED SPECIMEN
Reordered: 03/15/11 1529   Reorder Accession Number: 2915436

                    ****SPECIMEN CANCELLED****
Accn: 2915484   Acct: A1107400220
Spec: Blood   Collected: N/A
Priority: ROUTINE ROUNDS   Ord Phys: HOFF,LISA A

        Test Name: BILIRUBIN, DIRECT

        Cancelled: 03/16/11 0816   Cancelled by: Greene,Emma R
        Cancellation Reason: PENDING X1 DAY

                    ****SPECIMEN REJECTED****
Accn: 2915578   Acct: A1107400220
Spec: Blood   Collected: 03/16/11 0510
Priority: TIMED   Ord Phys: NANDLALL,BANEY P

        Test Name: CBC

        Rejected: 03/16/11 0756   Rejected by: MAK
        Rejection Reason: PLS RECHECK PER DEBRA
Reordered: 03/16/11 0756   Reorder Accession Number: 2916131

                    ****SPECIMEN CANCELLED****
Accn: 2915677   Acct: A1107400220
Spec: Blood   Collected: N/A
Priority: RTN AM   Ord Phys: LOPEZ,JOSE A

        Test Name: HEPATIC FUNCTION PANEL
                   CPK TOTAL
                   CBC

        Cancelled: 03/16/11 0229   Cancelled by:
        Cancellation Reason: ORDERED IN ERROR

M.R.Sherman,MD-LAB/T.Wentzell,MD-R.T.   EVERY,CHARLES
Health Central Laboratory   487530
Ocoee, FL 34761
** DO NOT DISCARD **   (M-02/24/30)
Discharge Cumulative Trend Report   Dr. NANDLALL,BANEY P

Patient Name: EVERY,CHARLES   Notification-Page 19
Med Rec #:   487530   Adm: 03/15/11
Dis Date   03/22/11
Phys-Service: NANDLALL,BANEY P - PROGESSIVE CARE
Acct #:   A1107400220
****

LABORATORY CANCELLED AND SPECIMEN REJECTED TESTS

****SPECIMEN CANCELLED****

Accn: 2916266   Acct: A1107400220
Spec: Blood   Collected: N/A
Priority: ROUTINE ROUNDS   Ord Phys: NANDLALL,BANEY P

        Test Name: CBC W/DIFF

        Cancelled: 03/16/11 1206   Cancelled by: KISHORE,CHRISTENA A
        Cancellation Reason: DONE

****SPECIMEN CANCELLED****

Accn: 2916535   Acct: A1107400220
Spec: Urine Random   Collected: N/A
Priority: ROUTINE ROUNDS   Ord Phys: ABREU,ELPIDIO A

        Test Name: LYTES WITH CREATININE/PROTEIN,
                   OSMOLALITY, URINE

        Cancelled: 03/16/11 1430   Cancelled by: SHEPARD,INDIRA B
        Cancellation Reason: DUPLICATE ORDER

****SPECIMEN CANCELLED****

Accn: 2918707   Acct: A1107400220
Spec: Blood   Collected: N/A
Priority: ROUTINE ROUNDS   Ord Phys: ROBERTSON,CECIL O

        Test Name: HEPATIC FUNCTION PANEL

        Cancelled: 03/18/11 1118   Cancelled by: KISHORE,CHRISTENA A
        Cancellation Reason: CMP ORDERED

****SPECIMEN CANCELLED****

Accn: 2918713   Acct: A1107400220
Spec: Blood   Collected: N/A
Priority: ROUTINE ROUNDS   Ord Phys: ROBERTSON,CECIL O

        Test Name: BASIC METABOLIC PANEL

        Cancelled: 03/18/11 1118   Cancelled by: KISHORE,CHRISTENA A
        Cancellation Reason: ORDERING CMP

M.R.Sherman,MD-LAB/T.Wentzell,MD-R.T.   EVERY,CHARLES
Health Central Laboratory   487530
Ocoee, FL 34761
** DO NOT DISCARD **   (M-02/24/30)
Discharge Cumulative Trend Report   Dr. NANDLALL,BANEY P

Patient Name: EVERY,CHARLES   Notification-Page 20
Med Rec #:   487530   Adm: 03/15/11
Dis Date   03/22/11
Phys-Service: NANDLALL,BANEY P - PROGESSIVE CARE
Acct #:   A1107400220
****

                  LABORATORY CANCELLED AND SPECIMEN REJECTED TESTS

                        ****SPECIMEN CANCELLED****
Accn: 2921344   Acct: A1107400220
Spec: Blood   Collected: N/A
Priority: RTN AM   Ord Phys: ROBERTSON,CECIL O

        Test Name: HEPATIC FUNCTION PANEL

        Cancelled: 03/21/11 1105   Cancelled by:
        Cancellation Reason: ORDERED IN ERROR
~~~~~~
                        ****SPECIMEN CANCELLED****
Accn: 2921448   Acct: A1107400220
Spec: Blood   Collected: N/A
Priority: TIMED   Ord Phys: NANDLALL,BANEY P

        Test Name: ALPHA-1-ANTITRYPSIN PHENO (2695

        Cancelled: 03/21/11 1143   Cancelled by: KISHORE,CHRISTENA A
        Cancellation Reason: ORDERED IN ERROR
~~~~~~

                            End of Report

M.R.Sherman,MD-LAB/T.Wentzell,MD-R.T.   EVERY,CHARLES
Health Central Laboratory   487530
Ocoee, FL 34761
** DO NOT DISCARD **   (M-02/24/30)
Discharge Cumulative Trend Report   Dr. NANDLALL,BANEY P

Patient Name: EVERY,CHARLES   Page 5
Med Rec #:   487530   Adm: 03/15/11
Dis Date   03/22/11
Phys-Service: NANDLALL,BANEY P - PROGESSIVE CARE
Acct #:   A1107400220
****

Accession Number	Test Name	Spec Type	Collection Date & Time	Status
2921533	ALPHA-1-ANTITRYPSIN (8161)	Blood	03/21/11 0408	Transmit
2921533	MITOCHONDRIAL AB, M2 (80008)	Blood	03/21/11 0408	Transmit
2921533	CERULOPLASMIN (800104)	Blood	03/21/11 0408	Transmit

                              End of Report
****

M.R.Sherman,MD-LAB/T.Wentzell,MD-R.T.   EVERY,CHARLES
Health Central Laboratory   487530
Ocoee, FL 34761
** DO NOT DISCARD **   (M-02/24/30)
Discharge Cum Incomplete Work Listing   Dr. NANDLALL,BANEY P

HEALTH CENTRAL HOSPITAL

DATE OF CONSULTATION: 03/16/2011

CONSULTING PHYSICIAN: CECIL ROBERTSON, M.D.

REFERRING PHYSICIAN: BANEY P. NANDLALL, M.D.

HEMATOLOGY CONSULTATION

REASON FOR CONSULTATION: Low platelets, anemia.

HISTORY OF THE CURRENT ILLNESS: The patient is an 91-year-old
man. Patient reports developing jaundice and dark urine and
complaining of dizziness. Patient states that three days ago he
was climbing out of his camper and he fell injuring his face, his
hand and his left leg. Patient now presents to the hospital with
severe jaundice and evidence for atrial fibrillation with rapid
ventricular response. Patient was found on evaluation to be
jaundiced, to have a total bili which is measured at 15.6, most
of it being direct bilirubin, with elevated AST, ALT and alkaline
phosphatase. Patient was also noted to have a very high CPK.
Patient was felt to be suffering from liver damage and to be in
rhabdomyolysis. Patient was noted also to be anemic with a
hemoglobin of 10.6 and to have low platelet counts. His platelet
count measured at 52,000. Hematology has been consulted to help
assist in the management of this patient who has liver damage and
rhabdomyolysis.

PAST MEDICAL AND SURGICAL HISTORY: The patient has a history of
coronary artery disease. Patient has had bypass surgery in the
past. He has hypertension, history of kidney stones and
hyperlipidemia.

MEDICATIONS: Home meds included metoprolol and Simvastatin.

LABORATORY DATA: He had a WBC of 6.5, hemoglobin of 10.6,
hematocrit of 32.2, platelet count of 52,000. Patient had a
total CPK of 1,305. Patient with a history of hypothyroidism,
had a TSH of 10.9. He had a total bilirubin of 15.6, and his
direct bili of 12, AST of 128, ALT of 107.

PHYSICAL EXAMINATION: VITAL SIGNS: On physical exam, patient
has a pulse of 83. Blood pressure 134/75, temp of 98.2. GENERAL
APPEARANCE: Patient was extremely jaundiced, awake and alert.
SKIN: Patient had severe bruising on the left side of his face,
bruises on his right hand and bruises on his left leg. LUNGS:
Bilateral breath sounds present. There is no wheezing, rales or
rhonchi at the time of my exam. CHEST: Patient has an old,
healed, midline thoracotomy scar. Cardiac appeared to be an

PATIENT: EVERY, CHARLES   ROOM: 220
ACCOUNT: 1107400220   VOICE ID: 00193691
MPI#: 487530
                                     Page 1

CONSULTATION

irregular rhythm at the time of my exam. ABDOMEN: Flat.
Patient has an old healed right lower quadrant scar. Abdomen is
soft, nontender. EXTREMITIES: Bruising on the left leg. No
pedal edema.

IMPRESSION: This is an 81-year-old man who has liver damage,
evidence for renal damage and he is in rhabdomyolysis, history of
taking a statin and of having a severe fall.

RECOMMENDATIONS: Patient should avoid statins at this time.
Patient is being treated with hydration and he is receiving other
supportive measures like antibiotics.

Would continue to hydrate the patient. Watch his total CPK.
Watch his BUN, creatinine and watch his liver function tests to
see if they improve, and patient should avoid Simvastatin.

CECIL ROBERTSON, M.D.

CR/04615309/ges
DD: 03/16/2011 23:29
DT: 03/17/2011 12:29
CC: BANEY P. NANDLALL, M.D.

PATIENT: EVERY, CHARLES   ROOM: 220
ACCOUNT: 1107400220   VOICE ID: 00193691
MPI#: 487530
                                         Page 2

                    CONSULTATION
Authenticated by CECIL O ROBERTSON MD 1881 On 03/17/2011 04:01:07 PM

HEALTH CENTRAL HOSPITAL

DATE OF ADMISSION: 03/15/2011

PRIMARY CARE PHYSICIAN: From out of town.

HISTORY OF PRESENT ILLNESS: This is a very pleasant 81-year-old
Caucasian male who is originally from Michigan. The patient stays
in the local area on an RV. He claims that he had a fall three
days ago and he did not remember the specific event and he thinks
he probably had syncope. Apparently, he was down for about an
hour and was unable to stand up. He had significant bruising in
the left periorbital and frontal area as well as some pain to the
left hip and some bruising to the right hand. He has been feeling
generally weak for at least about a week, having a poor appetite.
He has been nauseous but never vomited. He denies abdominal pain,
diarrhea, hematemesis, or melena. He has noticed some yellowish
skin discoloration for about three or four days.

PAST MEDICAL HISTORY: Includes dyslipidemia and coronary artery
disease, status post bypass.

HOME MEDICATIONS: Simvastatin, Metoprolol tartrate, unknown doses
for both.

ALLERGIES: UNKNOWN.

SOCIAL HISTORY: No tobacco, alcohol or drug abuse.

PAST SURGICAL HISTORY: Significant for appendectomy in the past.

FAMILY HISTORY: Noncontributory.

REVIEW OF SYSTEMS: The patient denies any weight loss, no night
sweats, no hematemesis, no melena, no headaches, no palpitations,
no abdominal pain, no lymphadenopathy, no polyuria.

PHYSICAL EXAMINATION:
VITAL SIGNS: Done in the emergency room shows the temperature to
be 97.2, heart rate 132, respiratory rate 22, pulse oximetry was
95% on room air, blood pressure was 116/63.
GENERAL APPEARANCE: The patient is a well-developed, well-
nourished male in no acute respiratory distress. He is obviously
having jaundice. He has a large hematoma to the left periorbital
and frontal areas. There is some mild bruising to the right
thumb. He is alert and awake and can provide adequate
information.
HEENT: Pupils are reactive to light. Conjunctivae were icteric,
but otherwise normal. _____ is clean and mildly dry.

PATIENT: EVERY, CHARLES   ROOM: 11
ACCOUNT: 1107400220   VOICE ID: 00193427
MPI#: 487530
                                       Page 1

                    HISTORY AND PHYSICAL

NECK: Supple.
LUNGS: Clear to auscultation.
HEART: Mildly tachycardic and irregular.
ABDOMEN: Flat and soft. There is mild epigastric tenderness. I did not appreciate any significant masses or organomegaly. No edema.

RADIOLOGIC STUDIES: There was a CT scan of the head, done without contrast by the emergency room which I do not have a formal report of, but as per the emergency room physician, Dr. Hoff, this was negative for acute intracranial abnormalities.

LABORATORY DATA: The latest CBC shows a white blood cell count of 11.6, hemoglobin of 12.9, platelet count is 61,000. INR was 1.04, BNP was 307, glucose was 118 with the BUN and creatinine of 27 and 1.7, total bilirubin was 15.6, calcium 9.0, alkaline phosphatase 225, AST 220, ALT of 107 with GFR of 41, lipase was 501, total CPK was 1,035. The urine has trace ketones and positive nitrates and a large amount of blood, trace leukocytes. TSH was 10.9.

ASSESSMENT AND PLAN:
1. Jaundice. A CT scan of the abdomen has been ordered, the results of which are pending.
2. Atrial fibrillation with episode of rapid ventricular response, initially he was placed on Cardizem drip and now the rate seems to be controlled. Will order a cardiology evaluation and will restart his beta blockers.
3. Coronary artery disease. Will obtain three sets of cardiac enzymes two more times q. 8 hours.
4. Hypothyroidism. At this point, will await cardiovascular evaluation before attempting to supplement this.
5. Urinary tract infection. Will start on ciprofloxacin 400 mg daily.
6. Rhabdomyolysis, probably due to trauma. Will give gentle fluid hydration.
7. Pancreatitis. Will await the CT scan of the abdomen and will order gentle fluid hydration.
8. Acute kidney injury, consider chronic kidney disease, probably hypovolemic in nature. Will await hydration and will repeat the labs in the morning.
9. Mild congestive heart failure, probably caused by episode of atrial fibrillation and rapid ventricular response.
10. Leukocytosis.
11. Thrombocytopenia.

JOSE A. LOPEZ, M.D.

PATIENT: EVERY, CHARLES   ROOM: 11
ACCOUNT: 1107400220   VOICE ID: 00193427
MPI#: 487530

Page 2

HISTORY AND PHYSICAL

JL/04545974/az
DD: 03/15/2011   17:00
DT: 03/15/2011   17:23

PATIENT: EVERY, CHARLES   ROOM: 11
ACCOUNT: 1107400220   VOICE ID: 00193427
MPI#: 487530
                                                Page 3

HISTORY AND PHYSICAL
Authenticated by JOSE A LOPEZ MD 5061 On 03/15/2011 06:15:39 PM

We recently received "This is Not a Bill" Explanation-of-Benefit papers for the cost of his nine days in the hospital in Florida at Health Central Hospital for the "side effects" of the drug companies "wonder" statin Drugs.

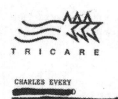

TRICARE EXPLANATION OF BENEFITS
Administered by: WPS TRICARE Administration
This is a statement of the action taken on your
TRICARE claim. Keep this notice for your records.

T R I C A R E

CHARLES EVERY

If you have questions about this notice, please call toll free at **1-866-773-0404**. For TDD, call **1-866-773-0405**. You can also visit us online at **www.tricare4u.com**

Date of Notice	04/25/2011
Summary of Claims Processed	FROM: 04/14/2011 TO: 04/21/2011
Sponsor SSN	XXX-XX-5805
Sponsor Name	Charles H Every
Patient Name	Charles Every

THIS IS NOT A BILL

Claim Number: 2011105 9767034
Provider #:   590660025 34761 0000
Provider Name: Health Central Hospital

Process Date: 04/21/2011

SERVICES PROVIDED BY	DATE OF SERVICE	AMOUNT BILLED	REMARKS
Health Central Hospital DRG standard 0441	03/15/11 - 03/22/11	$9,800.00	
Health Central Hospital DRG standard 0441	03/15/11 - 03/22/11	$2,712.20	
Health Central Hospital DRG standard 0441	03/15/11 - 03/22/11	$153.95	
Health Central Hospital DRG standard 0441	03/15/11 - 03/22/11	$28.00	
Health Central Hospital DRG standard 0441	03/15/11 - 03/22/11	$321.68	
Health Central Hospital DRG standard 0441	03/15/11 - 03/22/11	$9,541.93	
Health Central Hospital DRG standard 0441	03/15/11 - 03/22/11	$406.49	
Health Central Hospital DRG standard 0441	03/15/11 - 03/22/11	$2,083.00	
Health Central Hospital DRG standard 0441	03/15/11 - 03/22/11	$704.00	
Health Central Hospital DRG standard 0441	03/15/11 - 03/22/11	$113.00	
Health Central Hospital DRG standard 0441	03/15/11 - 03/22/11	$1,125.00	
Health Central Hospital DRG standard 0441	03/15/11 - 03/22/11	$290.00	
Health Central Hospital DRG standard 0441	03/15/11 - 03/22/11	$2,084.00	
Health Central Hospital DRG standard 0441	03/15/11 - 03/22/11	$2,547.00	

WPS
TRICARE FOR LIFE

Claim Number: 2011105 9767034   Process Date: 04/21/2011
Provider #:   590660025 34761 0000
Provider Name: Health Central Hospital

SERVICES PROVIDED BY	DATE OF SERVICE	AMOUNT BILLED	REMARKS
Health Central Hospital DRG standard 0441	03/15/11 - 03/22/11	$1,296.00	
Health Central Hospital DRG standard 0441	03/15/11 - 03/22/11	$130.00	
Health Central Hospital DRG standard 0441	03/15/11 - 03/22/11	$1,874.00	
Health Central Hospital DRG standard 0441	03/15/11 - 03/22/11	$2,315.00	
Health Central Hospital DRG standard 0441	03/15/11 - 03/22/11	$490.00	
Health Central Hospital DRG standard 0441	03/15/11 - 03/22/11	$972.00	
Total		$38,987.25	

CLAIM SUMMARY		BENEFICIARY SHARE	
TRICARE Amount Billed	$38,987.25	Cost Share/Copay	$0.00
TRICARE Allowed	$38,987.25	Deductible	$0.00
TRICARE Paid	$1,132.00		
Medicare/Other Ins. Paid	$9,964.41		

OUT OF POCKET EXPENSE:

	Beginning October 1, 2010		Beginning October 1, 2009		Beginning October 1, 2008	
	Limit	Met to Date	Limit	Met to Date	Limit	Met to Date
Catastrophic Cap	$3,800.00	$29.88	$3,000.00	$65.52	$3,000.00	$377.52

THIS IS NOT A BILL

Claim Number: 2011097 9872654   Process Date: 04/14/2011
Provider #:   593259553 32765 A001
Provider Name: Orlando Regional Healthcare

SERVICES PROVIDED BY	DATE OF SERVICE	AMOUNT BILLED	TRICARE ALLOWED	REMARKS
Orlando Regional Healthc 99222 - 1 MEDICAL OFFICE	03/16/11 - 03/16/11	$371.00	$136.05	106
Total		$371.00	$136.05	

CLAIM SUMMARY		BENEFICIARY SHARE	
TRICARE Amount Billed	$371.00	Cost Share/Copay	$0.00
TRICARE Allowed	$136.05	Deductible	$0.00
TRICARE Paid	$27.21		
Medicare/Other Ins. Paid	$108.84		

WPS
TRICARE FOR LIFE

OUT OF POCKET EXPENSE:

	Beginning October 1, 2010		Beginning October 1, 2009		Beginning October 1, 2008	
	Limit	Met to Date	Limit	Met to Date	Limit	Met to Date
Catastrophic Cap	$3,000.00	$20.88	$3,000.00	$65.52	$3,000.00	$377.52
Individual Deductible	$150.00	$0.00	$150.00	$0.00	$150.00	$32.89
Family Deductible	$300.00	$0.00	$300.00	$0.00	$300.00	$160.89

THIS IS NOT A BILL

Claim Number: 2011097 9872655   **Process Date:** 04/14/2011
Provider #: 593259553 32765 A001
Provider Name: Orlando Regional Healthcare

SERVICES PROVIDED BY	DATE OF SERVICE	AMOUNT BILLED	TRICARE ALLOWED	REMARKS
Orlando Regional Healthc	03/17/11 - 03/17/11	$201.00	$70.57	106
99232 - 1 MEDICAL OFFICE				
Total		$201.00	$70.57	

CLAIM SUMMARY		BENEFICIARY SHARE	
TRICARE Amount Billed	$201.00	Cost Share/Copay	$0.00
TRICARE Allowed	$70.57	Deductible	$0.00
TRICARE Paid	$14.11		
Medicare/Other Ins. Paid	$56.46		

OUT OF POCKET EXPENSE:

	Beginning October 1, 2010		Beginning October 1, 2009		Beginning October 1, 2008	
	Limit	Met to Date	Limit	Met to Date	Limit	Met to Date
Catastrophic Cap	$3,000.00	$20.88	$3,000.00	$65.52	$3,000.00	$377.52
Individual Deductible	$150.00	$0.00	$150.00	$0.00	$150.00	$32.89
Family Deductible	$300.00	$0.00	$300.00	$0.00	$300.00	$160.89

THIS IS NOT A BILL

Claim Number: 2011102 9939182   **Process Date:** 04/14/2011
Provider #: 593259553 32765 A001
Provider Name: Orlando Regional Healthcare

SERVICES PROVIDED BY	DATE OF SERVICE	AMOUNT BILLED	TRICARE ALLOWED	REMARKS
Orlando Regional Healthc	03/16/11 - 03/16/11	$214.00	$67.95	106
93306 - 1 ECHOCARDIOGRAPHY				
Total		$214.00	$67.95	

WPS
TRICARE FOR LIFE

CLAIM SUMMARY		BENEFICIARY SHARE	
TRICARE Amount Billed	$214.00	Cost Share/Copay	$0.00
TRICARE Allowed	$67.95	Deductible	$0.00
TRICARE Paid	$13.59		
Medicare/Other Ins. Paid	$54.36		

OUT OF POCKET EXPENSE:

	Beginning October 1, 2010		Beginning October 1, 2009		Beginning October 1, 2008	
	Limit	Met to Date	Limit	Met to Date	Limit	Met to Date
Catastrophic Cap	$3,000.00	$20.88	$3,000.00	$65.52	$3,000.00	$377.52
Individual Deductible	$150.00	$0.00	$150.00	$0.00	$150.00	$32.89
Family Deductible	$300.00	$0.00	$300.00	$0.00	$300.00	$160.89

THIS IS NOT A BILL

Claim Number: 2011103 9872584   Process Date: 04/14/2011
Provider #:   5935594333 34761 A001
Provider Name: Cecil Robertson

SERVICES PROVIDED BY	DATE OF SERVICE	AMOUNT BILLED	TRICARE ALLOWED	REMARKS
Cecil Robertson	03/22/11 - 03/22/11	$150.00	$101.48	106
99233 - 1 MEDICAL OFFICE				
Total		$150.00	$101.48	

CLAIM SUMMARY		BENEFICIARY SHARE	
TRICARE Amount Billed	$150.00	Cost Share/Copay	$0.00
TRICARE Allowed	$101.48	Deductible	$0.00
TRICARE Paid	$20.30		
Medicare/Other Ins. Paid	$81.18		

OUT OF POCKET EXPENSE:

	Beginning October 1, 2010		Beginning October 1, 2009		Beginning October 1, 2008	
	Limit	Met to Date	Limit	Met to Date	Limit	Met to Date
Catastrophic Cap	$3,000.00	$29.88	$3,000.00	$65.52	$3,000.00	$377.52
Individual Deductible	$150.00	$0.00	$150.00	$0.00	$150.00	$32.89
Family Deductible	$300.00	$0.00	$300.00	$0.00	$300.00	$160.89

THIS IS NOT A BILL

Claim Number: 2011103 9872505
Provider #: 593559433 34761 A001
Provider Name: Cecil Robertson

Process Date: 04/14/2011

SERVICES PROVIDED BY	DATE OF SERVICE	AMOUNT BILLED	TRICARE ALLOWED	REMARKS
Cecil Robertson 99223 - 1 MEDICAL OFFICE	03/16/11 - 03/16/11	$260.00	$198.99	106
Cecil Robertson 99233 - 1 MEDICAL OFFICE	03/17/11 - 03/17/11	$150.00	$101.48	106
Cecil Robertson 99233 - 1 MEDICAL OFFICE	03/18/11 - 03/18/11	$150.00	$101.48	106
Cecil Robertson 99233 - 1 MEDICAL OFFICE	03/19/11 - 03/19/11	$150.00	$101.48	106
Cecil Robertson 99233 - 1 MEDICAL OFFICE	03/20/11 - 03/20/11	$150.00	$101.48	106
Cecil Robertson 99233 - 1 MEDICAL OFFICE	03/21/11 - 03/21/11	$150.00	$101.48	106
Total		$1,010.00	$706.39	

CLAIM SUMMARY		BENEFICIARY SHARE	
TRICARE Amount Billed	$1,010.00	Cost Share/Copay	$0.00
TRICARE Allowed	$706.39	Deductible	$0.00
TRICARE Paid	$141.30		
Medicare/Other Ins. Paid	$565.09		

OUT OF POCKET EXPENSE:

	Beginning October 1, 2010		Beginning October 1, 2009		Beginning October 1, 2008	
	Limit	Met to Date	Limit	Met to Date	Limit	Met to Date
Catastrophic Cap	$3,000.00	$29.88	$3,000.00	$65.52	$3,000.00	$377.52
Individual Deductible	$150.00	$0.00	$150.00	$0.00	$150.00	$32.89
Family Deductible	$300.00	$0.00	$300.00	$0.00	$300.00	$160.89

THIS IS NOT A BILL

Claim Number: 2011103 9876495
Provider #: 591561574 34761 A001
Provider Name: Nephrology Assoc Of Central Florida

Process Date: 04/14/2011

SERVICES PROVIDED BY	DATE OF SERVICE	AMOUNT BILLED	TRICARE ALLOWED	REMARKS
Nephrology Assoc Of Cent 99222 - 1 MEDICAL OFFICE	03/16/11 - 03/16/11	$270.00	$136.05	106
Nephrology Assoc Of Cent 99233 - 1 MEDICAL OFFICE	03/17/11 - 03/17/11	$205.00	$101.48	106
Nephrology Assoc Of Cent 99232 - 1 MEDICAL OFFICE	03/18/11 - 03/18/11	$140.00	$70.57	106
Total		$615.00	$308.10	

WPS
TRICARE FOR LIFE

CLAIM SUMMARY		BENEFICIARY SHARE	
TRICARE Amount Billed	$615.00	Cost Share/Copay	$0.00
TRICARE Allowed	$308.10	Deductible	$0.00
TRICARE Paid	$61.62		
Medicare/Other Ins. Paid	$246.48		

OUT OF POCKET EXPENSE:

	Beginning October 1, 2010		Beginning October 1, 2009		Beginning October 1, 2008	
	Limit	Met to Date	Limit	Met to Date	Limit	Met to Date
Catastrophic Cap	$3,000.00	$29.88	$3,000.00	$65.52	$3,000.00	$377.52
Individual Deductible	$150.00	$0.00	$150.00	$0.00	$150.00	$32.89
Family Deductible	$300.00	$0.00	$300.00	$0.00	$300.00	$160.89

THIS IS NOT A BILL

Claim Number: 2011104 9853852   Process Date: 04/21/2011
Provider #:   591225842 34761 A001
Provider Name: **Medical Center Radiology**

SERVICES PROVIDED BY	DATE OF SERVICE	AMOUNT BILLED	TRICARE ALLOWED	REMARKS
Medical Center Radiology	03/17/11 - 03/17/11	$118.00	$35.95	106
93970 - 1 MEDICAL OFFICE				
Total		$118.00	$35.95	

CLAIM SUMMARY		BENEFICIARY SHARE	
TRICARE Amount Billed	$118.00	Cost Share/Copay	$0.00
TRICARE Allowed	$35.95	Deductible	$0.00
TRICARE Paid	$7.19		
Medicare/Other Ins. Paid	$28.76		

OUT OF POCKET EXPENSE:

	Beginning October 1, 2010		Beginning October 1, 2009		Beginning October 1, 2008	
	Limit	Met to Date	Limit	Met to Date	Limit	Met to Date
Catastrophic Cap	$3,000.00	$29.88	$3,000.00	$65.52	$3,000.00	$377.52
Individual Deductible	$150.00	$0.00	$150.00	$0.00	$150.00	$32.89
Family Deductible	$300.00	$0.00	$300.00	$0.00	$300.00	$160.89

WPS
TRICARE FOR LIFE

| THIS IS NOT A BILL |

Claim Number: 2011104 9853853   Process Date: 04/21/2011
Provider #: 591225842 34761 A001
Provider Name: Medical Center Radiology

SERVICES PROVIDED BY	DATE OF SERVICE	AMOUNT BILLED	TRICARE ALLOWED	REMARKS
Medical Center Radiology	03/16/11 - 03/16/11	$247.00	$73.95	106
74181 - 1 X-RAY				
Total		$247.00	$73.95	

CLAIM SUMMARY		BENEFICIARY SHARE	
TRICARE Amount Billed	$247.00	Cost Share/Copay	$0.00
TRICARE Allowed	$73.95	Deductible	$0.00
TRICARE Paid	$14.79		
Medicare/Other Ins. Paid	$59.16		

OUT OF POCKET EXPENSE:

	Beginning October 1, 2010		Beginning October 1, 2009		Beginning October 1, 2008	
	Limit	Met to Date	Limit	Met to Date	Limit	Met to Date
Catastrophic Cap	$3,000.00	$29.88	$3,000.00	$65.52	$3,000.00	$377.52
Individual Deductible	$150.00	$0.00	$150.00	$0.00	$150.00	$32.89
Family Deductible	$300.00	$0.00	$300.00	$0.00	$300.00	$160.89

| THIS IS NOT A BILL |

Claim Number: 2011104 9853854   Process Date: 04/21/2011
Provider #: 591225842 34761 A001
Provider Name: Medical Center Radiology

SERVICES PROVIDED BY	DATE OF SERVICE	AMOUNT BILLED	TRICARE ALLOWED	REMARKS
Medical Center Radiology	03/16/11 - 03/16/11	$77.00	$23.26	106
77074 - 1 34761				
Total		$77.00	$23.26	

CLAIM SUMMARY		BENEFICIARY SHARE	
TRICARE Amount Billed	$77.00	Cost Share/Copay	$0.00
TRICARE Allowed	$23.26	Deductible	$0.00
TRICARE Paid	$4.65		
Medicare/Other Ins. Paid	$18.61		

WPS
TRICARE FOR LIFE

OUT OF POCKET EXPENSE:

	Beginning October 1, 2010		Beginning October 1, 2009		Beginning October 1, 2008	
	Limit	Met to Date	Limit	Met to Date	Limit	Met to Date
Catastrophic Cap	$3,000.00	$29.88	$3,000.00	$65.52	$3,000.00	$377.52
Individual Deductible	$150.00	$0.00	$150.00	$0.00	$150.00	$32.89
Family Deductible	$300.00	$0.00	$300.00	$0.00	$300.00	$160.89

THIS IS NOT A BILL

Claim Number: 2011104 9853855   Process Date: 04/21/2011
Provider #:   591225842 34761 A001
Provider Name: Medical Center Radiology

SERVICES PROVIDED BY	DATE OF SERVICE	AMOUNT BILLED	TRICARE ALLOWED	REMARKS
Medical Center Radiology 74177 - 1 X-RAY	03/15/11 - 03/15/11	$335.00	$90.27	106
Total		$335.00	$90.27	

CLAIM SUMMARY		BENEFICIARY SHARE	
TRICARE Amount Billed	$335.00	Cost Share/Copay	$0.00
TRICARE Allowed	$90.27	Deductible	$0.00
TRICARE Paid	$18.05		
Medicare/Other Ins. Paid	$72.22		

OUT OF POCKET EXPENSE:

	Beginning October 1, 2010		Beginning October 1, 2009		Beginning October 1, 2008	
	Limit	Met to Date	Limit	Met to Date	Limit	Met to Date
Catastrophic Cap	$3,000.00	$29.88	$3,000.00	$65.52	$3,000.00	$377.52
Individual Deductible	$150.00	$0.00	$150.00	$0.00	$150.00	$32.89
Family Deductible	$300.00	$0.00	$300.00	$0.00	$300.00	$160.89

THIS IS NOT A BILL

Claim Number: 2011104 9853856   Process Date: 04/21/2011
Provider #:   591225842 34761 A001
Provider Name: Medical Center Radiology

SERVICES PROVIDED BY	DATE OF SERVICE	AMOUNT BILLED	TRICARE ALLOWED	REMARKS
Medical Center Radiology 71010 - 1 X-RAY	03/15/11 - 03/15/11	$32.00	$8.99	106
Medical Center Radiology 73510 - 1 X-RAY	03/15/11 - 03/15/11	$39.00	$12.12	106
Medical Center Radiology 70450 - 1 X-RAY	03/15/11 - 03/15/11	$144.00	$42.71	106
Total		$215.00	$63.82	

TRICARE FOR LIFE

CLAIM SUMMARY		BENEFICIARY SHARE	
TRICARE Amount Billed	$215.00	Cost Share/Copay	$0.00
TRICARE Allowed	$63.82	Deductible	$0.00
TRICARE Paid	$12.76		
Medicare/Other Ins. Paid	$51.06		

OUT OF POCKET EXPENSE:

	Beginning October 1, 2010		Beginning October 1, 2009		Beginning October 1, 2008	
	Limit	Met to Date	Limit	Met to Date	Limit	Met to Date
Catastrophic Cap	$3,000.00	$29.88	$3,000.00	$65.52	$3,000.00	$377.52
Individual Deductible	$150.00	$0.00	$150.00	$0.00	$150.00	$32.89
Family Deductible	$300.00	$0.00	$300.00	$0.00	$300.00	$160.89

THIS IS NOT A BILL

Claim Number: 2011105 9839998   Process Date: 04/21/2011
Provider #:   593269402 34761 A001
Provider Name: West Orlando Emerg Phys

SERVICES PROVIDED BY	DATE OF SERVICE	AMOUNT BILLED	TRICARE ALLOWED	REMARKS
West Orlando Emerg Phys	03/15/11 - 03/15/11	$688.00	$174.96	106
99285 - 1 MEDICAL OFFICE				
Total		$688.00	$174.96	

CLAIM SUMMARY		BENEFICIARY SHARE	
TRICARE Amount Billed	$688.00	Cost Share/Copay	$0.00
TRICARE Allowed	$174.96	Deductible	$0.00
TRICARE Paid	$34.99		
Medicare/Other Ins. Paid	$139.97		

OUT OF POCKET EXPENSE:

	Beginning October 1, 2010		Beginning October 1, 2009		Beginning October 1, 2008	
	Limit	Met to Date	Limit	Met to Date	Limit	Met to Date
Catastrophic Cap	$3,000.00	$29.88	$3,000.00	$65.52	$3,000.00	$377.52
Individual Deductible	$150.00	$0.00	$150.00	$0.00	$150.00	$32.89
Family Deductible	$300.00	$0.00	$300.00	$0.00	$300.00	$160.89

WPS
TRICARE FOR LIFE

THIS IS NOT A BILL

Claim Number: 2011105 9853991   Process Date: 04/21/2011
Provider #:   205689196 34761 A001
Provider Name: Mohammad R Mastali MD

SERVICES PROVIDED BY	DATE OF SERVICE	AMOUNT BILLED	TRICARE ALLOWED	REMARKS
Mohammad R Mastali MD 99214 - 1 MEDICAL OFFICE	03/25/11 - 03/25/11	$161.00	$103.28	106
Total		$161.00	$103.28	

CLAIM SUMMARY		BENEFICIARY SHARE	
TRICARE Amount Billed	$161.00	Cost Share/Copay	$0.00
TRICARE Allowed	$103.28	Deductible	$0.00
TRICARE Paid	$20.66		
Medicare/Other Ins. Paid	$82.62		

OUT OF POCKET EXPENSE:

	Beginning October 1, 2010		Beginning October 1, 2009		Beginning October 1, 2008	
	Limit	Met to Date	Limit	Met to Date	Limit	Met to Date
Catastrophic Cap	$3,000.00	$29.88	$3,000.00	$65.52	$3,000.00	$377.52
Individual Deductible	$150.00	$0.00	$150.00	$0.00	$150.00	$32.89
Family Deductible	$300.00	$0.00	$300.00	$0.00	$300.00	$166.89

Remark Codes:

Payment has been made to the provider of care for claim 2011105 9767034.
Did you know that TRICARE Explanation of Benefits are available on the website, TRICARE4u.com? As a registered user you have the ability to view any Explanation of Benefits. If you would like to become a registered user please visit us at TRICARE4u.com.
Payment has been made to the provider of care for claim 2011097 9872654.
Payment has been made to the provider of care for claim 2011097 9872655.
Payment has been made to the provider of care for claim 2011102 9939182.
Payment has been made to the provider of care for claim 2011103 9872504.
Payment has been made to the provider of care for claim 2011103 9872505.
Payment has been made to the provider of care for claim 2011103 9876495.
Payment has been made to the provider of care for claim 2011104 9853852.
Payment has been made to the provider of care for claim 2011104 9853853.
Payment has been made to the provider of care for claim 2011104 9853854.
Payment has been made to the provider of care for claim 2011104 9853855.
Payment has been made to the provider of care for claim 2011104 9853856.
Payment has been made to the provider of care for claim 2011105 9839998.
Payment has been made to the provider of care for claim 2011105 9853991.

106:    Tricare For Life is the secondary payer to Medicare and the amount allowed is Medicare's allowable. If you are not satisfied with the amount allowed, please contact your Medicare carrier for review. Any Medicare adjustment to their allowable will be sent to Tricare For Life by Medicare.

All TRICARE claims must be filed no later than one year after the date the services were provided or one year from the date of discharge for an inpatient admission for facility charges billed by the facility. Professional services billed by the facility must be submitted within one year from the date of service. For additional information please visit www.tricare4u.com.

WPS
TRICARE FOR LIFE

PAID TO	AMOUNT PAID	AMOUNT YOU OWE
MULTIPLE	$1,523.22	$0.00

IMPORTANT NOTICE

1. THIS NOTICE CAN BE USED:

A. As a deductible certificate to show your providers the amount of the outpatient deductible met as of the date of this notice.

B. As a record of bills paid or denied (if you submitted other medical expenses not shown on this form, you will receive a separate notice).

C. To collect other insurance. This notice may be used to claim benefits from a secondary insurance policy. Since the insurance company may keep this notice, it is advisable that you keep a record of this information.

IF YOU NEED MORE INFORMATION:

- Check your TRICARE handbook.
- See the Health Benefits Advisor or Health Care Finder at the nearest Uniformed Services medical facility.
- Always give your Sponsor's Social Security number when writing about your claim.
- If inquiring about this claim, please provide the claim number located on the front of this form.
- Contact us at the telephone number shown on the front of this form.
- Written inquiries except Appeals (see #4) and Grievances (see #10) should be mailed to the following address:

    WPS TRICARE
    P.O. Box 7889
    Madison, WI 53707-7889

2. TIME LIMIT FOR FILING CLAIMS:

Example:	For services received:	File Claims By:
	1 Jan 92-31 Dec 92	31 Dec 93
	1 Jan 93 & after	1 year after Date of Service

All claims for benefits submitted under CHAMPUS/CHAMPVA for dates of service prior to January 1, 1993 must be filed with the appropriate CHAMPUS contractor no later than December 31 of the calendar year immediately following the year in which the service or supply was provided. For services on and after January 1, 1993, all claims must be filed with the appropriate TRICARE contractor no later than one year from the date of service, or the date of discharge in the case of inpatient care.

If your claim was denied because it was not filed on time and you believe you were not at fault, contact us or your Health Benefits Advisor for assistance. In limited circumstances, exceptions may be made.

3. TYPE OF SERVICE CODES:

First Position:

A = Ambulatory surgery cost-shared as inpatient (Active duty family members only)
I = Inpatient
M = Outpatient maternity care cost-shared as inpatient
N = Outpatient cost-shared as inpatient
O = Outpatient Care Other
P = Outpatient partial psychiatric hospitalization care cost-shared as inpatient

Second Position:

1 = Medical Care
2 = Surgery
3 = Consultation
4 = Diagnostic/Therapeutic X-Ray
5 = Diagnostic Laboratory
6 = Radiation Therapy
7 = Anesthesia
8 = Assistance at Surgery
9 = Other Medical Service

A = DME Rental/Purchase
B = Drugs
C = Ambulatory Surgery
D = Hospice
E = Second Opinion on Elective Surgery
F = Maternity
G = Dental
H = Mental Health Care
I = Ambulance
J = Program for Persons with Disabilities

4. YOUR RIGHT TO APPEAL THIS INITIAL DETERMINATION:

If you disagree with the determination on your claim, you have the right to request a reconsideration. Your SIGNED written request must state the specific matter with which you disagree and MUST be mailed to the following address no later than ninety (90) days from the date of this notice. If the postmark on the envelope is not legible, then the date of receipt is deemed the date of filing. Include a copy of this notice. On receiving your request, all TRICARE claims for the entire course of treatment will be reviewed.

    WPS TRICARE
    ATTN: APPEALS
    P.O. Box 7490
    Madison, WI 53707-7490

5. IF PAYMENT NOT BASED ON THE FULL AMOUNT BILLED:

The amount TRICARE may pay is limited by law to the **lowest** of:

A. The CHAMPUS Maximum Allowable Charge; i.e. the charge made 80 percent of the time by physicians or suppliers in the country for similar services during the base year adjusted by where the services were rendered; or

B. Prevailing charge; i.e. the charge made 80 percent of the time by physicians or suppliers in the state for similar services during the base year; or

C. The amount the provider actually charges for the service or supply; or

D. The fiscal year 1988 prevailing charge adjusted by the Medicare Economic Index (MEI); or

E. The discounted charge that a provider has agreed to accept under a special program approved by the Director, TRICARE Management Activity.

6. PATIENT'S SHARE OF THE COST FOR AUTHORIZED CARE:

Inpatient Benefits   *See remarks on front.

Outpatient Benefits

Active duty family members of sponsor E-4 and below:	First $50 of allowable charges incurred by a patient each fiscal year (1 October-30 September) not to exceed $100 per family plus 20% of allowable charges after deductible has been paid.
Active duty family members of sponsor E-5 and above:	First $150 of allowable charges incurred by a patient each fiscal year (1 October-30 September) not to exceed $300 per family plus 20% of allowable charges after deductible has been paid.
Former spouses, Non-active duty members and their families:	First $150 of allowable charges incurred by a patient each fiscal year (1 October-30 September) not to exceed $300 per family plus 25% of allowable charges after deductible has been paid.

Claim payments are subject to the provision that the beneficiary cost-share is collected by the provider. The provider's failure to collect the cost-share can be considered a false claim and/or may result in reduction of payment.

7. SPONSOR, PATIENT, OR DEPENDENT NOT ENROLLED OR NOT ELIGIBLE ON DEERS:

If the Defense Enrollment Eligibility Reporting System (DEERS) indicates that the sponsor, patient and/or dependent is not enrolled or eligible for TRICARE benefits, you should contact your Health Benefits Advisor or your service personnel office. Future claims will be denied if you are not enrolled in DEERS. If the claim was denied and the sponsor has recently gone on the patient's identification (ID) card or parent's ID for dependent children under 10 years of age. If the sponsor is retired, resubmit the claim with the sponsor's retirement papers and a photocopy of the patient's (ID) card. If the sponsor is deceased, report to any service personnel office to get enrolled or call the appropriate number listed below.

8. IDENTIFICATION CARD (ID) OR ELIGIBILITY EXPIRED ON DEERS:

The Defense Enrollment Eligibility Reporting System (DEERS) indicates that the patient's ID card or eligibility has expired. To get a new ID card or extend eligibility, if sponsor is active duty, report at once to any parent service personnel office; if sponsor is retired or deceased, contact any service personnel office. If the claim was denied, when the patient obtains a current ID card, resubmit the claim with a photocopy of the new ID card (both front and back sides). In an emergency, call the appropriate number listed below.

FOR DEERS INFORMATION CALL:	
CALIFORNIA 1-800-334-4162	HAWAII & ALASKA . 1-800-527-5602
ALL OTHER STATES	1-800-538-9552

9. BENEFICIARY NOTICE:

Please review the services shown on the front side of this TRICARE Explanation of Benefits. If you find that payment consideration has been made for any services that you did not receive, or that services were provided by a health care professional that you did not see, please call the FRAUD AND ABUSE number at 1-866-773-0404.

10. TO FILE A GRIEVANCE:

If you are dissatisfied with the ability of WPS personnel to provide appropriate health care services, access to care, timeliness of care, quality of care or service, or level of care or service, you may file a grievance. Mail your written grievance with supporting information to:

    WPS TRICARE
    ATTN: Priority / Grievances
    P.O. Box 8974
    Madison, WI 53708-8974

TRICARE

CHARLES EVERY
7377 CURRIE RD
NORTHVILLE MI 48168-4816

If you have questions about this notice,
please call toll free at 1-866-773-0404. For
TDD, call 1-866-773-0405. You can also visit
us online at www.tricare4u.com

TRICARE EXPLANATION OF BENEFITS
Administered by: WPS TRICARE Administration
This is a statement of the action taken on your
TRICARE claim. Keep this notice for your records.

Date of Notice	04/25/2011
Summary of	FROM: 04/13/2011
Claims Processed	TO: 04/13/2011
Sponsor SSN	XXX-XX-5805
Sponsor Name	Charles H Every
Patient Name	Charles Every

THIS IS NOT A BILL

Claim Number: 2011095 2799846   Process Date: 04/13/2011
Provider #:   383316559 48103 B001
Provider Name: Ann Arbor Family Practice

SERVICES PROVIDED BY	DATE OF SERVICE	AMOUNT BILLED	TRICARE ALLOWED	REMARKS
Ann Arbor Family Practie	11/12/10 - 11/12/10	$113.00	$73.12	106
99238 - 1 MEDICAL OFFICE				
Total		$113.00	$73.12	

CLAIM SUMMARY		BENEFICIARY SHARE	
TRICARE Amount Billed	$113.00	Cost Share/Copay	$0.00
TRICARE Allowed	$73.12	Deductible	$0.00
TRICARE Paid	$14.62		
Medicare/Other Ins. Paid	$58.50		

OUT OF POCKET EXPENSE:

	Beginning October 1, 2010		Beginning October 1, 2009		Beginning October 1, 2008	
	Limit	Met to Date	Limit	Met to Date	Limit	Met to Date
Catastrophic Cap	$3,000.00	$20.88	$3,000.00	$65.52	$3,000.00	$377.52
Individual Deductible	$150.00	$0.00	$150.00	$0.00	$150.00	$32.89
Family Deductible	$300.00	$0.00	$300.00	$0.00	$300.00	$160.89

THIS IS NOT A BILL

Claim Number: 2011102 9932768   Process Date: 04/13/2011
Provider #:   650641688 32809 D001
Provider Name: Ameripath Florida Llc

SERVICES PROVIDED BY	DATE OF SERVICE	AMOUNT BILLED	TRICARE ALLOWED	REMARKS
Ameripath Florida Llc 88185 - 19 LAB WORK	03/16/11 - 03/16/11	$1,539.00	$936.70	106
Ameripath Florida Llc 88184 - 1 LAB WORK	03/16/11 - 03/16/11	$163.00	$82.13	106
Ameripath Florida Llc 88182 - 1 LAB WORK	03/16/11 - 03/16/11	$207.09	$0.00	301
Ameripath Florida Llc 88185 - 4 LAB WORK	03/16/11 - 03/16/11	$324.00	$197.20	106
Total		$2,233.09	$1,216.03	

CLAIM SUMMARY		BENEFICIARY SHARE	
TRICARE Amount Billed	$2,233.09	Cost Share/Copay	$0.00
TRICARE Allowed	$1,216.03	Deductible	$0.00
TRICARE Paid	$243.21		
Medicare/Other Ins. Paid	$972.82		

OUT OF POCKET EXPENSE:

	Beginning October 1, 2010		Beginning October 1, 2009		Beginning October 1, 2008	
	Limit	Met to Date	Limit	Met to Date	Limit	Met to Date
Catastrophic Cap	$3,000.00	$20.88	$3,000.00	$65.52	$3,000.00	$377.52
Individual Deductible	$150.00	$0.00	$150.00	$0.00	$150.00	$32.89
Family Deductible	$300.00	$0.00	$300.00	$0.00	$300.00	$160.89

Remark Codes:

Payment has been made to the provider of care for claim 2011095 2799846.

Did you know that TRICARE Explanation of Benefits are available on the website. TRICARE4u.com? As a registered user you have the ability to view any Explanation of Benefits. If you would like to become a registered user please visit us at TRICARE4u.com.

Payment has been made to the provider of care for claim 2011102 9932768.

106:    Tricare For Life is the secondary payer to Medicare and the amount allowed is Medicare's allowable. If you are not satisfied with the amount allowed, please contact your Medicare carrier for review. Any Medicare adjustment to their allowable will be sent to Tricare For Life by Medicare.

301:    Medicare has applied the following provider cut-back, discount, or other payment reduction to claim 2011102 9932768 (THE DIAGNOSIS IS INCONSISTENT WITH THE PROCEDURE.). Neither the beneficiary, nor TRICARE For Life is obligated to pay this amount.

All TRICARE claims must be filed no later than one year after the date the services were provided or one year from the date of discharge for an inpatient admission for facility charges billed by the facility. Professional services billed by the facility must be submitted within one year from the date of service. For additional information please visit www.tricare4u.com.

PAID TO	AMOUNT PAID	AMOUNT YOU OWE
MULTIPLE	$257.83	$0.00

$6,121.00
38,987.25
$45,108.25 Totals

WPS.
TRICARE FOR LIFE

If we do get billed for some of the costs that Medicare or our insurance company will not cover, shouldn't we be able to send them to the pharmaceutical company that made the drug and the FDA that approve it? None of his health problems were the result of anything he did on his own.

The subject of medical costs remind me of a book that Dr. Cicel B. Jackson, MD of Garden City, MI had on the shelf in his waiting room (years ago, at the time of one of my pregnancies) *It's Cheaper to Die*. He said he got it from his father as a joke. Could any of his patients have felt like leaving when they noticed the book? Knowing what the costs are for a stay in the hospital or even just a visit to your doctor, the book's title may be truer now than we'd like to think.

Famous people that we have probably all heard about, like, Lucile Ball, Sam Walton (one of the richest people in the world), Lou Gerhig, Michael Landon, Elizabeth Edwards, Farrah Fawcett, Elizabeth Taylor, Paul Newman, Dave Thomas (founder of Wendy's), Steve Jobs (founder of Apple Computer) and so many others, that "couldn't" be saved, even with all their money, by anything available through the traditional doctors, surgery, or drugs (poisons)! I believe that conventional AMA doctors are committing murder and don't even realize it because of their lack of knowledge of vitamins, minerals, and herbs—God-given cures.

I used to wonder why some of the alternative doctors or scientist didn't try to reach these people and let them know what could save their lives. Then I found out that Robert Barefoot did try to reach some of them, but security was so tight, he couldn't get thru to them. This may certainly be the case with others that may have tried to reach these people.

These famous and wealthy individuals probably had what was known as "the very best doctors in the world" because they could afford them. But what good did all their money do for their health? They surely would have given all that they had, don't you think? But real cures from God's nature—herbs, vitamins, minerals—are kept secret from the doctor's knowledge. What a very sad and inexcusable state of affairs.

We absolutely need to change this waste of human life—the sooner the better for everyone.

1   St. Germain Chiropractic, P.A. office, 877 S. Orange Blossom Trail, Apopka, FL

2   "Library of Food and Vitamin Cures" by Dr. Jonathan V. Wright, MD, "Report #7-The Miricle Mineral" Pages 77

3   "The Douglass Report" by William Campbell II, MD, Volume 12 Number 2, June 2012, Pages 4-6

4   http://www.cdc.gov/dhdsp/data_statistics/fact_sheets/docs/_fs_heart_disease.pdf Page

5   "Media Says: No Cure for heart disease" by William Faloon, Life Extension—Sept. 2010 Pages 7-9

6   "Natural Healing" newletter (Subber 2011) by Dr. Mark Stergler Page 2 "According to the Dietary Supplement Health Education Act of 1994, supplement makers are forbidden from claiming that any of their products can cure or even prevent any illness or disease."

7   "Nutritution and Healing" by Jonathon V. Wright Page 82

8   "Real Cures" newsletter Volume 7, Number 7 by Dr. Frank Shallenberger, Page 7 (Review of the JUPITER study published in "Archives of Internal Medicine" (review exposed the statin myth. There is absolutely no advantage with statins)

9   "How Mainstream Medicine BREAKS your Heart" by William Campbell Douglass II, MD found in "The Douglass Report", Page 1

10 "The Douglass Report" by Dr. William Campbell II, MD Page 9 "The 10 hidden and forbidden Cures that will save your life"

11 http://www.wxyz.com/dpp/news/health/do-the-side-effects-of-statins-outweigh-their-benefits

12 Second Opinion, P.O. Box 8051, Norcross, GA. 30091-8051. 800-262-3164 or 770-399-5617. www.secondopinionnewsletter.com

13 "Second Opinion" by Dr. Robert J. Rowen

14 "World's Dumbest Supplements Myths" by Dr. David G. Williams Page 18

Chapter Four

ARE WE STILL IN THE DARK AGES?

Those people that still believe the FDA is there to protect and help the general public are really in the dark ages! This may have been the original intent, but obviously it isn't even close to that now! Money has gotten in the way and seems to be primarily what they are protecting, rather than citizens' health.

Many people have killed for money, but they usually end up in jail. Pharmaceutical companies, the FDA, the AMA, and doctors kill people with drugs (poisons), and surgeries, but get away with it. After all, they have the licenses to do it.

More on the "Wonder Drugs"

Years ago, when I was just a kid, I heard my parents tell of my great aunt and uncle's baby, who died of scurvy. None of the drugs or other doctors' treatments could save his life. Now we know that vitamin C would have saved the baby from scurvy. This is another sickness caused by a lack of nutrition and the medical doctor's ignorance!

When I was somewhat older, an uncle died of cancer, regardless of all the chemo treatments he had undergone. I remember my aunt saying, "If we had known how sick the chemo would make him, we never would have agreed to the treatments!" The chemo did not help him one little bit, he died without having one "good" day. It is doubtful that the chemo extended his life whatsoever. Perhaps it even shortened it? The chemo certainly killed his immune system!

A few years ago, my only sister also died of cancer. She went through chemo and was on oxygen, yet suffered for two years before passing. I don't recall her having even one good day in those two years, either.

I was with her during one of her treatments. The liquid that was being used as the base in her chemo treatments was alcohol. My sister did not drink any alcoholic beverages, and as a result, became drunk. With all this liquid in her, she needed to use the restroom. She got up and headed for the restroom, not realizing she was attached to the IV holder. I jumped up to escort her with the IV. When we reached the bathroom door, she turned to me and said, with quite a slurred voice, "You can come in the bathroom with me, 'cause we're related . . . but *he* (the IV) has to stay out!"

She and my brother-in-law lived with us for about six months while she received treatments at a hospital in the Detroit area. After six months she really wanted to go home to Michigan's Upper Peninsula. She continued more chemo treatments there. When she left the Detroit-area hospital she was still alive and therefore counted as a "cancer survivor." So the "cancer survivor" statistics can be quite misleading!

Unfortunately, at the time they lived with us, we did not know about the cancer cures of vitamin C, Coral Calcium Complete, wheat germ extract, or any of the other cancer-curing plants and herbs. We gave her some coral calcium that we had on hand, and it seemed to help some, along with a diet rich in vegetables and fruits (when she could keep them down.) The small amount of coral calcium we were giving her wasn't nearly enough, as we learned later.

My husband did come up with a drink that she could keep down, which contained "Boost" that she was told to drink, protein power, eggs, and a few other nutrients.

My brother-in-law had diabetes and died a little over a year later. His and my sister's diet was terrible. They ate lots of sweets (desserts and candy), deep-fried foods, and few vegetables, fruits, or vitamins. He also carried a very large bag (from Sam's Club) of M&M's in his brief case. They often ate at fast food places and mostly after my sister became ill, because he didn't know how to cook.)

My brother-in-law had type two diabetes, which usually affects middle-aged people. Approximately ninety percent of diabetics are type two. Many of these people are overweight and inactive. Type one diabetes or juvenile diabetes usually affects people before the age of twenty.

A friend at church also had cancer. He died even though he went through chemotherapy. He only hung on for a few months. Was he, perhaps, luckier than the others since he didn't suffer as long?

We have had other friends and relatives that had cancer, submitted to the chemo treatments, and still died. They also endured a great deal of misery during their chemotherapy. The loss of all their hair, nausea, loss of appetite, weight loss, depression, loss of energy and so on. There are enough "side" effects to make you feel like you wish it were "all over" already.

There are scores of alternative doctors that have cured cancer victims with certain vitamins and minerals (many with vitamin C, Calcium, plants, and herbs). Treating cancer through nutrition makes you start feeling better almost immediately. But why should the AMA and the FDA bother to listen to these alternative doctors? There is no really big money in it since they can't patent vitamins, minerals, or plants, which are considered foods.

The big pharmaceutical companies have tried to patent vitamins. This is one thing that they have failed to accomplish! In fact, there are countries in Europe whose governments have taken vitamins off the shelves and made them available only via prescription. If we don't do something now, could we be next

We may be hearing more in the future about the "dangers of nutritional supplements" by big pharma and its big government allies. When have you ever heard of deaths caused by taking food supplements?

Big pharma is still trying to turn some of the high-potency vitamins and minerals into prescription drugs. Luckily, there are some US senators and representatives that are willing to prohibit the FDA from obtaining federal funds to establish and enforce these regulations.

Dr. Julian Whitaker, MD[1] of the Wellness Institute has compiled a sample letter for people to write to various government officials, it follows:

Dear Senator
(Congressman/woman, FDA commissioner):

Re: Draft Guidance for Industry: Dietary Supplements, New Dietary Ingredient Notifications, and Related Issues.

The FDA's proposed regulations for dietary supplements are onerous, unnecessary, and would do horrific damage to me, my family, and the country. Furthermore, the FDA's intentions are counter to the letter and spirit of DSHEA, which became law seventeen years ago.

I urge you and your colleagues to uphold this law and force the FDA to stop this illegal activity. My freedom of choice and my access to nutritional supplements, which my family and I depend on, are at stake.

Sincerely,

The people that have been cured of Cancer are few and far between. Even with the poor record of results, the medical profession still continues to use antiquated methods to try to cure cancer (and many other illnesses.)

I like what Albert Einstein said, "Great spirits have always encountered violent opposition from mediocre minds." Maybe proponents of the AMA and the FDA have consumed too much of their own products—they are certainly mind-boggled!

I know only a couple of cancer survivors, at least one of whom did not have chemo.

Personally, if I found out that I had cancer I would never agree to do chemotherapy. Chemo kills all of your immune system, the same immune system you need to fight disease or infection. The idea behind chemo is that although it kills your immune system, it will also kill the cancer. But what is left to fight any other illnesses? In other words, doctors hope that chemotherapy kills the cancer before it kills you!

TABLE: US CANCER DEATHS
(Source: The American Cancer Society)

YEAR	DEATHS[2][3]
1975	-428,151
1980	-470,213
1985	-502,801
1990	-536,515
1995	-558,895
2000	-560,821
2005	-545,884
2009	-530,988

In prostate cancer alone, one death occurs every 15 minutes. This equals four deaths per hour, and times twenty-four hours in a day means there are ninety-six prostate-cancer-related deaths every day. With 365 days in a year that adds up to 35,040 deaths every year. Keep in mind, this is for one type of cancer that affects men only.

After all these years, and billions of dollars spent on finding a cure, the death rates from cancer have not decreased, but have significantly increased annually. No pharmaceutical cure has been found by the AMA or "big pharma," but they haven't decreased their begging for more and more money to keep searching.

The Pfizer Drug Company came out with a new drug for pancreatic cancer, which was approved by the FDA and brought in over one billion dollars in sales in 2010. And, yet, I haven't heard anything on the news about this wonder drug actually curing cancer. Have you?

I have also wondered how wearing a pink ribbon is supposed to help cure cancer. It is intended to promote "cancer awareness," but who isn't aware of cancer? We probably all have relatives or friends who have or have had cancer. Of course, selling those pink ribbons does bring in a lot of money.

After all these years and all the drugs that have not cured any diseases, the medical industry is still concocting worthless drugs!

Albert Einstein's definition of insanity is "doing the same thing over and over and expecting different results."

I have read in some of our Health news letters that over eighty percent of Doctors in the United States have said that they would *not* submit themselves or their families to chemotherapy. In Canada, over ninety percent of doctors have said they would *not* submit themselves or their families to this type of treatment. Is there something they know that they are not telling their patients? Why aren't they? Could it be related to money?

A woman is being sued for "murder" because she stopped taking her son for his chemo treatments. The chemo was making him so sick that he pleaded with his mother to not make him take any more treatments. Apparently what treatments he did receive weren't much help; he died. The authorities now blame the mother for his death. I haven't heard how her court case came out. I've been thinking that if she were acquitted, the FDA might not want this information to come to the public's attention.

There is a Dr. Lorraine Day, MD[4], who is known worldwide for her work with AIDs patients. She went along with all the recommended

AMA treatments, until she, herself got cancer. Then she searched online and found many alternative cures for cancer! She found out that there was a considerable amount of research that had been held back and was therefore unknown to most conventional doctors. As a result, she refused to undergo surgery, chemotherapy, radiation or any of the usual medical treatments, much to the disagreements of her fellow physicians. Dr. Day eventually cured herself through nutrition.

My husband and I own her videos, *Cancer Doesn't Scare Me Anymore* and *You Can't Improve On God*. How about that—a doctor, an MD, using nutrition instead of medical procedures!

These videos are probably still available. Call 1-800-556-4846 or write ITV Direct, Inc., P.O. Box 7083, Beverly, MA 01915.

Maybe the health food and grocery stores have made a little money from Dr Day, but medical institutions, the pharmaceutical industry, and the FDA certainly did not.

Of heart disease, which was discussed earlier, the AMA and Pharmaceutical Industry claim "they have not cured, but have helped with drugs and surgery." Helped whom? Both drugs and surgery brings in billions of dollars every year. There are a half-million people in America who die from heart attacks every year.

Doctors now say that blood pressure should be only 110/70. How and why do you suppose the decrease came about? Ideal blood pressure used to be 120/80. People who used to be normal are now in need of medications. It sure is helping to increase the revenue of drug manufacturers.

We were all given a conscience (that small, internal voice) to know right from wrong, provided we do not willfully disregard it. It certainly appears that money yelled so loud that big pharma, the FDA, medical schools, and other members of the medical community have totally lost their good conscience!

A good alternative doctor or chiropractor might recommend you purchase lecithin, selenium, magnesium, zinc, or other supplements. How many dollars do you think this will put in their pockets? They may never be paid with a lot of money, but will be paid in knowing how much good they did for someone's health. This will do wonders for their conscience and the good feelings they get about being able to really help people get well and feeling good. You can't put a price tag on these rewards. So, money doesn't seem to be the incentive for alternative doctors or chiropractors.

I will opt for a good alternative Doctor or chiropractor any time!

You should be able to find alternative doctors near you on the internet. Here are a couple of sites you can start with:

American Board of Clinical Metal Toxicology, www.abcmt.org

International College of Integrative Medicine, www.icimed.com

You may have to seek a good Chiropractor on your own. You can talk to friends and family that use a chiropractor that they like, or take a trial-and-error approach.

For instance, my right jaw was out of place for over a year, which made for difficult eating. I went to one chiropractor for several visits. It felt like he was trying to jerk my head off. He suggested trying different heights in pillows at night, which did help a little. After several visits, I tried another chiropractor, who my husband and I still both use. With only one visit, and a very gentle adjustment, the jaw is just fine.

On the subject of a doctor's occupation being called a "practice," when I was just a small child, I had several ear aches. Some could have been the result of having allergies and blowing my nose often (and hard), causing fluid to back up into my ears. After all, the eyes, ears and nose are all connected. The doctor lanced my ears several times. He also said I would probably be hard of hearing when I got older. Today I *am* very hard of hearing. I'm legally deaf in my left ear and the right ear isn't much better. This is probably because of all the scar tissue resulting from all the surgical lancing of my ears. The younger doctors of today haven't even heard of ear lancing. Apparently the doctors of years ago were just "practicing" again.

There are supplements available now that are helping improve some age-related hearing loss. Hearing aids today also have some remarkable technology and are more than just amplifiers. There is also some phenomenal surgery available to restorer hearing, but it is, unfortunately, very expensive. It starts at $30,000 per ear.

[1]   Dr. Julian Whitaker, MD Director or the Whitaker Wellness Institute, Newport Beach, CA

[2]   http://seer.cancer.gov/csr/1975_2009_pops09/browse_csr.php?section=2&page=sect_02_table.06.html

[3]   http://www.multpl.com/united-states-population/table
Note: Taking information from the above two websites to get the information in the table.

[4]   "Cancer doesn't scare me anymore" Video by Dr. Lorraine Day, MD published by ITAV Direct, Inc, PO Box 7083, Beverly, MA 01915 (800-556-4846)

Chapter Five

YOU ARE WHAT YOU EAT!

God makes real nutrition that is much better for us than any man-made mess! There are stories of countless numbers of people recovering from common and even life threatening diseases by nutrition—Foods—vitamins—minerals—herbs.

For instance, here are a couple of homemade remedies for the common cold and sore throat.

Cough Syrup:

Take the skin off an onion. Cut it in half and then cut each half into fairly thin slices. Separate the onion rings from each slice and put in a bowl. Next, cover the onion slices in the bowl with honey. (The amount of honey depends on the size of the onion used.)

Let the onion and honey sit over night. The honey should become a thinner consistency, like syrup. Drain the syrup from the onion slices and pour in a bottle. Your cough syrup is now ready for use.

For a sore throat:

Make salsa! Dip with nachos or other whole grain chips—we like the Sun Chips. We found this out some years ago when we went with our children and grandchildren to a Mexican restaurant. I had one of the worst sore throats I'd ever had. The grand kids kept insisting I try the restaurant's great salsa. I kept thinking it would really wreak havoc on the sore throat. With their continual orders, "You've got to try it!" I put just a touch on a teaspoon and ate it. To my amazement the salsa made the sore throat feel better than it had felt in days. So, I continued to indulge! We now use the salsa "fix" for any sore throat,—which we seldom get.

As mentioned early in this book, chiropractors learn a lot on nutrition in their eight years of education. There are many alternative doctors that have gone out on their own and studied and practice nutrition. These alternative doctors are fully aware they are going against what they were taught in medical schools and against the powerful AMA and FDA.

Because of their nutritional knowledge, these doctors for nature cures have had their offices raided and records confiscated. One such doctor was Jonathan V. Wright, MD of Frederic, MD. Two dozen heavily armed people kicked the door down to his office and even stuck a revolver to some of his workers' heads. For two hours they were held at gun point. These people were wearing government badges! They were sent to Dr. Wright's office by the FDA. What horrible offense was he committing? He was prescribing vitamins. Two federal grand juries didn't, or couldn't, return an indictment.[1]

In 1984, Dr. Carl Reich and Robert R. Barefoot have done much research regarding calcium and curing cancer. [2][3]

Below I summarize a recent article from HSI (Health Science Institute):

The Native Americans from the North had a cancer cure that was nearly lost forever, until the following. Mrs. A. had considerable pain in her right breast for some years before she finally went to Toronto, Canada to see if the doctors there could find out the cause. Before she left, an old Ojibwe Indian she knew told her it was cancer and he could cure her. She went to the doctors in the city anyway. They wanted to remove the breast, but she refused. She remembered what the old Indian had said and thought she should give his herbs a try.

Some years later she told her story to the head nurse at the Providence Hospital in Ontario, Rene Caisse, and gave her the same formula, with the four herbs, she had received from the Ojibwe

Indian. A few years later a favorite aunt of Rene's was diagnosed with cancer and was given only six months to live. Rene was allowed to try the herbal medicine and the aunt lived for another twenty-one years.

In the mean time, word had spread about the cancer cure and more and more people came to the clinic that Rene eventually opened. The name of the herbal medicine cancer cure was Essiac.

In spite of a petition signed by eight doctors, the Department of Health and Welfare in Ottawa arrested her for "practicing medicine without a license" in an attempt to silence her. This was just the beginning of her troubles. Even though 387 of her cured patients would testify on her behalf, fewer than fifty were called on. The officials claimed their testimonies were "invalid." She was threatened with heavy fines, imprisonment, harassed, and brought before a special cancer commission.

Her clinic was closed in 1942. She passionately protected the herbal formula and would only turn it over if assured it would not be hidden away for the benefit of the conventional treatments. In 1977, she sold the formula to The Resperin Corp. of Toronto for one dollar. The witness of the contract signing was John F. Kennedy's personal physician, Dr. Charles Brusch. He had been one of the supporters of Nurse Rene Caisse's work. He used Rene's native formula successfully in his own fight against bowel cancer.

The miraculous herb formula for Essiac was finally revealed; it contains burdock root, Indian rhubarb, sheep sorrel, and slippery elm in very strict amounts, which are carefully blended. But the fight to shut down the use of this proven cancer cure was not over. The Canadian government closed the Resperin's tests in 1982. [4]

In 2004 and 2006 more tests, finally allowed, of the Essiac herb formula were done, and this time, with some very favorable results. "So powerful it literally flushes cancer out of the body!" You can get Essiac but be very careful of buying imitations! [4]

To purchase Essiac:

Essiac Canada International, www.vitaminshoppe.com. One 10.5 oz. bottle is US $25.07. The Vitamin Shoppe has a 30-day return policy. Please see the website for details.

For thousands of years, herbs have been used for healing by the Egyptians, Chinese, Native American Indians, and other cultures.

There are some conventional AMA Doctors that have learned of some of these cures using nutrition, vitamins, minerals, and herbs, but are afraid to apply this knowledge. The fear of losing their licenses stops them. What a very sad state of injustice.

In the nineteenth century, tens of thousands of women were dying every year from Puerperal "childbed" fever. This epidemic was the result of doctors performing autopsies and then doing vaginal exams with their hands still contaminated with decomposing tissues. Midwives had a much lower rate of childbed fever than the doctors.

Dr. Ignaz Semmnelweis, knowing the better survival rate of midwives, required the doctors in his department to wash their hands with a disinfectant. Death rates immediately dropped to only 1.3%.[5]

When he realized the great importance of washing hands he tried, many times, to persuade the other doctors, but was ignored or met with hostility. After these many attempts to promote the washing of hands, Dr. Semmnelweis was committed to an insane asylum. He was only forty-seven years old when he died there.

How many public bathrooms do you go into now, where you will see a sign that reads: "Employees must wash hands before returning to work"? At least, in this case, we've come a little way out of the dark ages.

Linus C. Pauling, the Nobel Prize-winning scientist, forty years ago, discovered intravenous vitamin C therapy of high doses was a remarkable anti-cancer agent. He was ridiculed by the medical establishment, which also tried to destroy his reputation by claiming he was senile. [6]

Could it be that cancer was generating billions in revenue? And if this cancer cure were widely known, it would ruin the medical industry's "goldmine" and possibly tarnish its reputation through its willful concealment of cancer cures.

We might have had a difficult time believing the above stories about doctor's Offices being raided and some doctors losing their licenses, because we believe that all doctors intend to help people get well.

In 2003? My husband, Chuck and I spent our three months in South Carolina, we were going to an alternative doctor, Dr. James Shortt, for chelation treatments. This was our second year seeing him. He and a nurse told us about their office recently being raided by armed thugs wearing government badges, who forced them out of their office. These pistol bearing goons proceeded to take his files and whatever else they wanted.

He was currently in the process of being tried in a Medical building Court! Having had some very good results with his treatments, we were interested in testifying on his behalf. We, several others of his patients, and other Doctor friends went to court. When we arrived at the building we were ushered to a room on the second floor. After a considerable time, one of the doctors said, "You know, we're just being hidden out of sight, Let's go downstairs to the lobby and get noticed." So, that is what we all did.

None of us were ever asked to testify or even allowed into the court room!

Some years ago, when we were visiting my sister and her husband at their winter home in Alabama (near the Florida border) they told us about sitting next to a doctor from Florida while they were having chelation therapy.

They asked the doctor why he didn't get the chelation therapy in Florida, since it was also available there. He replied, "I can't. I'm the head of the AMA in Florida."

Chelation therapy, for those who are not familiar with it, is a means of unclogging your arteries. It is an alternative to bypass surgery. Chelation is derived from the Greek word "chele," or claw. Chelation therapy is a man-made amino acid that is put in an IV bag and slowly administered intravenously into the body over a period of one to three hours. This process circulates through 60,000 miles of blood vessels and is done under the supervision of a doctor. The chelation therapy attracts certain substances, usually metal atoms like lead, mercury, cadmium, etc. that are eliminated thru the kidneys as part of one's urine within the following 24 hours. A liquid Roto-Rooter[7], so to speak.

Most people seem to be of the opinion, "If it's worth knowing about my Doctor would know about it!" If only this could be true. Prayerfully, in the future, doctors will be taught in their 8 years of study about the real cures of nutrition, herbs, minerals and some from very ordinary plants.

Linus Pauling did more than just discover the all powerful vitamin C that earned him the Nobel Prize in 1937. (This same doctor also discovered removal of 328 mg of phytosterols from wheat germ increased cholesterol absorption by 43%, which reduces the risk of heart disease) [8]

But this amazing discovery has been ignored (deliberately) by big wigs of the Drug Industry that aren't even interested in anything that doesn't fill their pockets with big bucks. They are zealously bent on killing cancer cells (and our immune systems) with chemo and radiation with all the horrendous side effects!

If we would stick with eating more natural foods that we often can grow ourselves, or perhaps purchase from local farm markets, we will be a lot better off than filling our bodies with the man made messes and their side effects.

The man made mess may be quick and easy to use, but many are quick to get us sick and can earn us some long term bad health issues. (These fake foods with little or no nutrition in them)

Just keep in mind—You are what you eat and put in/on (like the "patch") your body.

---

[1]   "Shocking Midical Coverups" by Matthew Simmons. Copyright 2010 by Healthier News, LLC, page 6-7

[2]   "The Disease Conspiracy" by Robert R. Barefoot, Page 73-90, printed by RGM Management Services, LLC

[3]   http://barefootscureamerica.com/191-2/

4   Health Science Institute Newletter "Member Alert" Article "Discovered. A Cancer Killing Miricle from the Forzen North . . . almost lost forever" Page 4 by Michele Cagan Note: A monthly publication—not dated which we received early 2011

5   "Life Extension" newsletter by Dr. Eric Braverman, MD (Director of Path Medical, New York, NY), Page 2

6   Cameron E. and Pauling, L. Cancer and Vitamin C: A Discussion of the Nature, Causes, Prevention, and Treatment of Cancer With Special Reference to the Value of Vitamin C (Camino Books) ISBN 0-940159-21-X

7   Roto-Rooter™ is used to unclog plumbing by professional plumbers http://www.rotorooter.com

8   http://lpi.oregonstate.edu/infocenter/phytochemicals/sterols/

Chapter Six

OBESITY AND DIET

Obesity is another really big money maker for the pharmaceutical industry!

With a good portion of the American population being obese, this is like the pharmaceutical industry having a golden goose. This subject of obesity could also have been included in chapter two "Follow the Money!" However, so many people are affected with this "disease" that it merits a chapter of its own.

In 2008, 147 Billion Dollars are spent annually on medical-related products for obesity. [1] Obese people are a major target for drugs to treat an endless number of obesity-related illnesses. This means more and more money for the pharmaceutical industry.

There was an article in the January 2011 issue of *Reader's Digest* by award-winning, science journalist, Gary Taubes, entitled, "Is This Any Way to Lose Weight?" It was accompanied by a picture of two eggs and bacon arranged on a plate in a smiley face.

He explains why conventional diets do not work and what to eat to lose weight that will work. It could be that the right fats (natural fats from animals—like beef and dairy products) can be your best friend while certain carbohydrates are your worst enemy. The so-called low-fat diet promoted by the American Heart Association is actually bad for your heart. [2]

My husband and I showed this article to our chiropractor, Dr. D. W. Brockenshire, Chiropractic Physician, Applied Kinesiologist, and Clinical Nutritionist in Plymouth, Michigan, to get his opinion. He exclaimed, "That's what I eat for breakfast"!

Gary Taubes, has also written a book called *Why We Get Fat and What to Do About It*." Mr. Taubes's book can get a bit technical, but he has the ability to explain everything in down-to-earth language with some very good examples and pictures, too. Not only is it understandable, it proves many of the long-held beliefs that many of us have, although they have never been proven. We think they make sense and most everyone says they are true—including so-called authorities. The "calories in, calories out" theory is a perfect example.

Most processed foods do not come naturally low in fat. Man has to mess with them in some way to make them low-fat. This is just another case where the more man messes with something, the more it will mess you up! The low fat diets that we are told to eat for heart health are actually bad for your heart.

My husband and I are examples of what a vegetarian, low-fat diet can do to ruin your health, because we ate this way for years. We followed what the so-called experts recommended!

All of the examples of my husband's heart problems, which I talked about earlier, happened while on the diet recommended by the American Heart Association, among other "authorities."

I also experienced health problems while on this diet. I had Intermittent claudication (a painful cramping of leg muscles because of poor circulation). I could only walk twenty to twenty-five steps at a time before having to stop because of the pain. Going uphill or up any stairway was horrible. This kept getting worse and worse until I thought I would eventually need a wheelchair to get anywhere without pain. At the time, we did not relate these problems to diet.

Some years back, I went to the doctor and had a standard blood test done. The following day his office called and wanted me to come back for another test. The doctor didn't believe the results.

But the first test was right—I was very anemic! He asked if I'd had any fainting spells. I hadn't, but I had noticed my skin seemed very pale. I thought I just needed to get out in the sun more.

I was sent straight to the hospital, where I received four blood transfusions! Still, I never related the problem to diet.

Another problem I had was that my fingers were getting out of shape; they bent in weird angles and had lumpy knots on the joints. I was also getting varicose veins on the back of my right leg.

It finally hit me during my husband's last heart problem. You are what you eat!

This is when we finally began looking into books and getting newsletters from alternative doctors for the answers to our health problems. We have found a wealth of good knowledge and information that has been most favorable health-wise!

Census statistics show that vegetarians die younger. Reports from Pediatric Adolescent Medicine conclude vegetarian children have "impaired psychomotor development." Furthermore, "vegetarian teens use laxatives more often than non-vegetarians." [3][4]

Another powerful article states that "vegetarians in a research done at the University of Massachusetts medical school linked their diets to slumping sex function and muscle loss as well as some bone damage."[5]

Just a thought: have you ever heard any Centenarian say being a vegetarian was even a part of the reason for their long life?

For nearly fifty years we have been told that in order to lose weight we need to consider the ratio of calories we take in (food) and calories we put out (exercise) This idea sounds logical and appears to make sense. One of the problems with this theory, however, is that it has never been proven. There have been no real scientific studies to test this theory. Apparently it sounded right to many people, as everyone seems to have bought into it—myself included.

Did you ever get on an exercise machine that showed how many calories you were burning? A single slice of bread is over 100 calories. How much time on an exercise machine does it take to just burn 100 calories?

I'm not indicating exercise is worthless; your whole body needs exercise, especially your heart. But exercise is not the key to losing weight. If it were, why do we weigh less in the morning when we get up (after lying in bed all night) then we do in the evening (after being active all day)?

We have a friend that underwent bypass surgery several months ago. He just eats and sits or sleeps all day—no exercise. I saw him just recently and he is so thin, he looks emaciated! So if "calories in and calories out" is accurate, why isn't he overweight?

Also, with this theory of "calories in and calories out," it shouldn't matter what you eat. Does a pound of candy have the same nutritional value as a pound of other food? What we eat makes all the difference. As I mentioned earlier Gary Taubes's book is a great eye opener. A low-carbohydrate diet is key, not a low-fat diet. Say goodbye to white flour, sugar, pastas, starchy vegetables, and hello to real butter, whipped cream, bacon, eggs, meat, cheese, leafy greens, tomatoes, and other vegetables rich in nutrients.

Not only are these foods much tastier than any low-fat, man-made messes, but they are better for your health and your heart. You will lose more weight and keep it off. You will not feel hungry like you do on more traditional diets and you will require fewer of the drugs that cost you a fortune. And when you stop the diet and restart the drugs, the weight will come right back on—and then some.

Dr. Robert C. Atkins had it right, all along. His "diet" has now been proven to be healthier, too.

The general manager of Health & Science, Ben Harder, said at *U.S. News and World Report*, "For the paleo diet, additional evidence is needed to show conclusively whether or not it is as effective as some people hypothesize." In other words, they already have some "evidence" it works. [6][7]

The paleo diet certainly sounds like the diets recommended by Dr. Atkins and Gary Taubes in his book, *Why We Get Fat and What to Do About It*.

Dr. William Campbell Douglas II, MD said he knows of people that have beaten rheumatoid arthritis, multiple sclerosis (MS), GERD, and more by eating these foods.

This way of eating is easy to follow. It is tastier, requires no calorie-counting, and is easy to keep the weight off. Try it . . . You'll like it!

All the symptoms of intermittent claudication disappeared. No more anemia! My fingers are actually straightening out and the varicose vein troubles are a thing of the past! I am living proof that this diet, along with lots of calcium and vitamin C, works!

I actually feel much better now at eighty than I did in my sixties! When I was in my sixties, I started having the varying health problems on the American Heart Association Diet.

I have more energy and can do more things because I feel like doing them. For instance, I used to hire professional carpet cleaning companies to clean our carpet because my legs hurt so much whenever I would try to do the work myself. Now I use a carpet cleaning machine and do the work myself! (Would you like to hire me? Just joking—I'm too busy now. Today I brushed on a wood sealer on our deck and tomorrow I'll apply some weather proof varnish on it.)

Another problem I was having, started in 1954 when I was seven months pregnant with our first child. My husband was in the Air Force and was sent to Biloxi, Mississippi for training. My ankles and feet swelled so much I couldn't wear any of my regular shoes. I had to get some bigger shoes and slippers.

There were several of the Air Force wives that were pregnant at the same time I was and only four Air Force doctors were assigned to all these pregnant women. The office had about three rows of ten chairs per row. The women in the first seats in the first row were the first to see the doctors. As one of the doors in one of the doctor's offices opened and a woman left, the next in line went into that office, and so on. As the women went in, we all moved forward. It was like the game of musical chairs.

With this game of musical chairs, we never seemed to see the same doctor two times in a row. This also meant that we never knew ahead of the visit which doctor we would be seeing.

The doctors on the base were concerned that I might have toxemia. They sent me to the hospital where I stayed for five days of treatment. This meant mainly that my feet were elevated and I was on an 800-calories-a-day diet! The doctor's claimed the swelling was because of the salt air from the ocean. I don't know what the diet was for, because I was anything but overweight.

It was only natural to think when I got back to Michigan that the swelling would stop. It didn't. The swelling continued, particularly in the summer months.

When I was pregnant with our second child, Dr. C.B. Jackson said to take alfalfa tablets. He said they were a natural diuretic and he didn't want to put me on a medication while I was pregnant. Perhaps he was close to what we now call an alternative doctor. The alfalfa tablets did help quite a bit, but there was still some swelling, mainly during the summer. Last year all the stores that used to sell the alfalfa pills, stopped carrying them.

When we started taking quite a few of the vitamin C tablets, the swelling of my ankles and feet stopped. I don't just mean that the "C's" helped a lot, I mean the swelling completely stopped! I was amazed at how thin my ankles became. I don't ever remember them being this thin! I'm thrilled—this was another unexpected, pleasant surprise from vitamin C.

But back to the alfalfa tablets: I recommended alfalfa to a relative last year (when we could still buy it), and gave him some of my alfalfa pills to try. He recently had started having problems with swollen feet (edema). His wife, (a registered nurse) asked how many he should take and what the side effects would be if he happened to take too many.

I told them to take whatever he needed to take to reduce the swelling. I said, "I take two— one in the morning and one in the evening. alfalfa is classified as a food. What happens to a farm animal, such as a cow, if it eats too much alfalfa? There are no side effects!"

I was tempted to say that one of the side effects was that he might "moo" or that he might dry up and float away!" I, contained myself, however, and held my tongue.

He was taking a diuretic prescription that was giving him some unwanted side effects. He later said he not only liked the alfalfa better than the drug he was taking, but the alfalfa worked much better on his swelling.

When the alfalfa pills became unavailable, I told him about the even better results the vitamin C was yielding. I also showed him and his wife my wonderful skinny ankles. I told him I was taking at least six per day in addition to some of the chewable kind. My husband and I don't know if they have tried the vitamin C tablets or not. Maybe I should ask him to raise his pant leg, so we can find out?

We do take lots of vitamins now, but we take the most of vitamin C, and the mineral, Coral Calcium Complete.

And all the bad press that the egg has gotten lately is a "yolk"! A major study of 800,000 people has proven that people who eat eggs live longer and have fewer heart attacks than those who do not. Eggs are another good source of vitamin D. [8]

Eggs are rich in protein and other nutrients that help one to feel full longer. With more and more studies on eggs, researchers are finding more and more benefits to be had from the lowly egg! The egg yolks (that we have been told to avoid) contain two amino acids that have major antioxidant ingredients, even more than an apple or several cranberries! A research team has discovered that egg proteins are converted by the enzymes in the stomach and small intestines to produce peptides that act like ACE inhibitors, which lower blood pressure. The search goes on and that little, ole "bad egg" can even help prevent heart disease and cancer!

Bring on the fat.

The body needs fats, but you can't expect the American Heart Association to say they have been wrong all at once. But they *are* doing it little by little, bit by bit. You are now being told that you need omega three fatty acids and fish oil and it is good to cook with olive oil. Well, it is a start.

The Eskimos are fat lovers. It's a big part of their diets. Eskimos have almost no coronary heart disease. Studies also show that other groups of people (in other countries), with few heart diseases, also consume a lot of fat! [9] So I repeat, "go ahead and have your steak, hamburger, eggs, cheese, whipped cream, and real butter (a good source of vitamin K). These are all heart healthy! (Are there any vitamins or minerals found naturally in any of the advertisements of "heart healthy," man-made spreads (messes)? Fiber is good, especially when obtained from nature's own vegetables and fruits. Fiber can be found in lots of those leafy green salads.

The things to avoid are the bad carbohydrates, like white bread (or anything from white flour), other starchy foods, and sugars. Sugars are really bad for you! Whole grain foods should be eaten in moderation, unless you are very skinny.

An excellent sweetener to use is stevia. Stevia is an herb and much sweeter than sugar. Just a little goes a long way. It used to be available only in health food stores, but I have been seeing it lately in some regular grocery stores.

It is easier to prescribe drugs than it is to change a person's diet. There isn't any money in trying to improve a person's eating habits. Besides, most conventional doctors have very little knowledge about nutrition.

Last year I started noticing cinnamon capsules in the vitamin sections in several stores. My husband and I wondered when cinnamon became a vitamin. What makes cinnamon so special? Shouldn't it be in the baking isle where the rest of the spices are?

Then we heard the story of a diabetic man that went to his regular doctor's appointment to have his regular blood work done. He told the doctor that he just ate a big piece of apple pie and that his blood sugar would probably be very high. The doctor thought his blood sugar should be very high, too. But his blood sugar was actually in the normal range!

This was a really big surprise to both of them and one for which the doctor had no explanation! Out of curiosity the doctor did a lot of research and testing. In 2000 a study published by the USDA itself, cinnamon demonstrated the greatest ability to stimulate healthy cellular glucose metabolism. It can even help your body keep strong and natural insulin levels. [10]

No wonder cinnamon is in capsule form in the vitamin section of stores. Now we know why it is there and what good the spice cinnamon can do for you.

[1]   http://www.healthy.arkansas.gov/programsServices/chronicDisease/ Documents/WorksiteWellness/WorksiteWellnessPresentation.pdf

[2]   "Is This Any Way to Lose Weight?" by Gary Taubes in Reader's Digest Jan., 2011

[3]   "Pediatric Adolescents Medicine" page 7 Fall 2010

[4]   "Had Enough" page 7 booklet by Dr. William Campbell Douglass II, MD Fall, 2010

[5]   "Had Enough" page 7 booklet by Dr. William Campbell Douglass II, MD Fall, 2010

[6]   "The Douglass Report" by Dr. William Campbell Douglass II, MD Sept., 2011 No 5 page 3-5

[7]   "Eat these Lose Weight" Reader's Digest magazine Jan. 2011 pages 110-119

[8]   "Had Enough" page 21 booklet by Dr. William Campbell Douglass II, MD Fall, 2010

[9]   http://www.livestrong.com/article/450725-eskimo-diet-heart-disease/

[10]   http://www.ncbi.nlm.nih.gov/pmc/articles/PMC2901047/

Chapter Seven

COLLOIDAL SILVER AND HYDROGEN PEROXIDE

Have you ever heard of colloidal silver? It is a potentially life-saving, infection-fighting liquid. It has saved more lives from deadly infections, since its discovery over ninety years ago, than any other natural substance in existence!

At Syracuse University, Dr. Robert O. Becker, M.D. and his colleagues proved that colloidal silver kills many of the deadly microorganisms that are no longer affected by prescription drugs. [1] Colloidal silver further demonstrated over 650 different disease-causing pathogens are killed by it within a few minutes. Dr. Cesar Garcia Ramirez in Mexico is using it on their AIDS patients with amazingly good results. [2][3]

The outstanding, life-saving results of colloidal silver are endless! So why haven't most people heard about it?

The FDA has ruled that people who sell and make colloidal silver cannot tell people about its amazing infection fighting powers of this proven, all natural, safe liquid! Hundreds of studies in those ninety years in medical universities in both the United States and Europe, have substantiated the great infection-killing qualities of colloidal silver. In 1999, the FDA placed severe restrictions on what can be put on labels of colloidal silver. It can only be described as a "mineral supplement". If colloidal silver is represented as anything more, the offending manufactures can be shut down and their inventory confiscated. And the FDA has followed through on this threat.

If any of you saw the "blue man" on TV, he totally misused colloidal silver. Several people saw him, including our doctor, who knows my husband and I use colloidal silver, and couldn't pass up the chance to tell us about him. I can't imagine how much colloidal silver he could possibly take to make himself blue! We take some colloidal silver every day. Could he possibly been taking something else, too, like blue food coloring?

Chuck and I use colloidal silver every day, and wouldn't be caught without it. We add about an eye dropper full to many of our drinks, which are usually water. We have a small spray bottle in our bathroom and give a few sprays in our mouths, particularly if we think we might be getting a sore throat. Even if your mouth just feels a bit dry, give it a couple squirts of the colloidal silver.

Our grandkids love it when we spray any bug bites, cuts, scrapes, or sun burns with colloidal silver. We also place a dash of it in the water for washing fruits and vegetables. Its good uses go on and on.

Perhaps some of you might remember your grandmother placing a silver spoon in the bucket of milk from her cow to keep the milk from spoiling?

I used to purchase colloidal silver from the Puritan's Pride Company at $36.00 for a four-ounce bottle, although it is now discontinued. Recently I saw, at one of the health food stores, a gallon bottle of "silver water" for forty dollars! I now make my own for less than one dollar per quart! The colloidal silver we make is better than what we used to buy. There is a laser light that comes with equipment for making your own colloidal silver. Without using the light, the colloidal silver looks just like plain water. With the light you can detect the minute silver particles. What we made contained more silver than what we purchased.

We bought our equipment to make colloidal silver through a dentist who is retired and now lives in Arizona. We have run across another source in a book about it, *The Ultimate Colloidal Silver Manual*, and supplies for making your own colloidal silver. We do not know the costs, but purchasing colloidal silver (if you can even find it) can be very expensive. The company's contact information is:

Life and Health Research Group, LLC
P.O. Box 1239
Peoria, AZ 85380-1239
Phone: 1-888-846-9029

HYDROGEN PEROXIDE (oxygen)

You can live for a few weeks without food. You can live for days without water, but without Oxygen hardly even a few minutes. Oxygen is the most essential element we need to live! To fight infections, your body's cells actually produce hydrogen peroxide to fight off the invaders.

The human body is composed of approximately 75% water (by weight) is approximately 90% oxygen. Nothing is more important to your health than Oxygen.

Hydrogen Peroxide has been used in several foreign countries to heal nearly any known disease for well over 150 years. Here in the United States it has been nearly hidden from public knowledge. "Follow the Money" again—it costs only about 2 cents a day for daily maintenance. Hydrogen Peroxide (oxygen) may be about the most important information in this book.

For starting the Hydrogen Peroxide healing program, start with 3 to 4 drops in approximately 7 to 8 ounces of distilled water, taken 3 times per day (preferably on an empty stomach). Then for about 3 weeks, start adding 1 additional drop per day. At the end of this time you will be up to about 24 drops per day. You may encounter several bowel movements, especially in the beginning, while the body is detoxifying of many toxins. [1]

After this cleansing period go on the maintenance program of 3 t0 4 drops of Hydrogen Peroxide in 7 to 8 ounces of distilled water, 3 times per day. You will probably be amazed at how good, and how well you will feel.

Hydrogen Peroxide is NOT the kind that is purchased in the Drug store. This is 30% Food Grade—H2O2. This is very potent, and you would not want to put it full strength directly on your skin. It would hurt for a while (feels like a burn) and temporarily leaves the skin white. It is known as a "Strong Oxidizer".

To be more comfortable to the hands this food grade Hydrogen Peroxide needs to be diluted with 10 to 12 parts water to 1 part Peroxide.

Kill germs on counters, help prevent foot and nail fungus, remove mold and mildew, disinfect baby's pacifier and toys, boost laundry detergent power—etc. etc.

It's also good to add a little to the water for washing vegetables and fruits. It is great for adding to the water in your swimming pools. It's certainly much healthier than what pool companies sell you to put in your pools. Remember your body absorbs what is put on it. That is why "The Patch" has been so prominent for things like pain, stop smoking and so forth.

We found our food grade hydrogen peroxide on the internet at: www.dfwx.com/usage.html and www.dfwx.com/answers.html/

---

1   http://www.thesilveredge.com/pioneers.shtml

2   http://www.happyherbalist.com/aidsandhiv.htm

3   "The Colloidal Silver Conspiracy" pamphlet by Life & health Research Group, LLC

4   "The One Minute Cure" by Madison Cavanaugh published by Think-Outside the Book publishing, Inc by Page 74

Chapter Eight

A MERRY HEART— ANOTHER NATURAL CURE

"A merry heart doeth good, like a medicine" (Proverbs 17:22).

Some years ago a leading television personality, Virginia Graham, was diagnosed with cancer and was given little time to live. She read this scripture and decided to give it a try. She got all the funny videos and joke books she could find. She decided that even if she did die, she would at least "die laughing." Well, she did not die. She not only lived to tell her story (on her TV show), she also continued her TV show for several more years, until she retired.

There is an article called, "LAUGHTER IS GOOD MEDICINE" by Robert Brody (Longevity Dec.'88) on a study of laughter.

I have come across a more recent article in Bottom Line's book "Hushed-up 100" copyright 2012 by Broardroom Inc. Report #4 "Amazing! Laughter Lowers Cholesterol" by a Dr. Lee Berk MD, of Loma Linda University and Dr. Stanley Tan MD of Oak Crest Research Institute. They claim the study of the healing power of Laughter is still too new to know how much laughter to recommend. Apparently they did not know about the study by Mr. Brody back in 1988. Actually Laughter for healing goes all the way back to biblical times—"A **merry heart** doeth good like a **medicine**" How could you "over dose" on laughter? In my humble opinion—"The more, the "Better"!

Laughter is known to have healing results in heart health, blood pressure, diabetic patients, lowers cholesterol, inflammation and stress. I've never heard of a single medication that can have a favorable effect on such a large number of health related ills! The only side effects on laughing that I've heard anyone complain of is, "I laughed so hard, my stomach hurts."

Laughter is a great NATURAL medicine! You might even say—It's a "funny way to get well!" Most people would happily take this kind of "medicine" any time.

Will laughter and a sense of humor help us to live longer? How about "A laugh a day keeps the doctor away"?

Norman Cousins was once diagnosed with having a crippling spinal disease and was given a 1-in-500 chance for survival. Instead of accepting the pain killing drugs he substituted regular belly laughs. He completely recovered in just a few years. He has written a book, "Anatomy of an Illness" that might make some people take a second look at laughter in curing an illness.

Laughter is also electrochemical. It evidently lowers levels of hormones called catecholamines, responsible for arousal and alertness. These hormones include epinephrine, norepinephrine, and dopamine. A recent study at California's Loma Linda University Medical Center revealed that "laughter may be an anlogonist to the classical stress response" according to immunologist Dr. Lee S. Berk. Five subjects watched a sixty-minute humor video tape and five did not. Blood samples were taken every ten minutes for two hours, before, during and after the video. Epinephrine and dopamine levels in those who watched the video were significantly lower throughout.

Researchers speculate that laughter stimulates the pituitary gland to release endorphins and enkephalins, natural painkillers and chemical cousins to opiates such as Morphine and heroin.

Serving as organic analgesics, such chemicals may combat arthritis and other painful inflammatory conditions.

Laughter may reinforce our immune systems as well. A belly laugh could prompt the brain to block the manufacture of immune suppressants such as cortisone, says Berk. Recent studies show that laughter increases secretions of salivary immune-globulin (S-IgA)

Laughter may improve circulation, too. When the heart is activated, so is blood flow in the arteries and veins. Laughter can thereby speed the passage of oxygen and nutrients to cells. Arteries quickly expand and contract. Your systolic blood pressure can shoot from a norm of 120 to 200 during a major laugh, then briefly drop below its regular baseline, stimulating blood circulation. Laughter, with its stimulus-relaxation pattern could prove therapeutic against high blood pressure.

Breathing also benefits. As you laugh air gusts into your trachea as fast as 70 mph, cleaning mucus on the walls of your windpipe. Abruptly, but briefly interrupting normal breathing. Laughter cleans out foreign matter and helps stop bacteria from multiplying.

In laughing, we also seem to secrete enzymes that aid digestion. One reason hotels in the Catskills originally hired comedians was that management thought that laughter, in addition to seltzer, helped customers' digestion.

By distracting you from day-to-day concerns and banishing gloomy thoughts, if only for a moment. Laughter can relieve tension, boredom, and anxiety. Laughing is like uncorking a bottle of champagne—it takes the pressure off us so we can bubble over. It defuses anger and alleviates depression by implication, it can prevent heart attacks and cut the risk of cancer.

What counts more than an occasional mechanical laugh, however, is an enduring sense of humor. Medical authorities believe that only laughter derived from a true sense of the ridiculous is likely to exert lasting health benefits. Humor therefore, is no quick fix, no silver bullet.

"You simply have to consider what prevents longevity in the first place," says Fry, "Without laughter, I'm sure people would get sick more often and more severely. You can't laugh away the natural aging process. But you can minimize its consequences."

Wouldn't it be great if all doctors and nurses were trained in how to tell jokes and funny stories? What a marvelous way to help patients recover! How about being able to watch funny videos or DVDs on the hospital's televisions?

My husband and I don't think we ever heard about any doctors recently telling anyone to get a funny joke book or a humorous DVD and to have a good hard belly laugh instead of writing a prescription. Maybe doctors are not aware of all the good a generous belly laugh can do. They certainly wouldn't be taught about this in medical school. If they were, it would be a laugh!

Here are some Good Medicine Laughter jokes:

Oh, did you hear the one about the Walmart greeter?

The elderly lady that heard Walmart was hiring senior citizens as greeters? She applied for the job and was hired, but her job lasted for less than two hours. It seems a woman came in and was yelling and screaming all kinds of obscenities and lewd remarks at the two children that were with her.

The greeter said, "Welcome to Walmart, ma'am. Those are two lovely children you have. Are they twins?'

The woman replied, "No! They are not twins. One is seven and the other is ten. Are you blind, or just stupid?"

The greeter answered, "No, Ma'am. I'm neither blind nor stupid. I just can't understand why any man would want to go to bed with you two times!"

The supervisor then told the greeter, "Sorry, but I don't think you're cut out for this job."

How about this one?

One Sunday afternoon a young couple with a little, four-year-old son, was talking with their neighbor. The young couple had recently moved to this rural area from the city. The young wife said to her neighbor, "This morning I saw a strange animal in our back yard. I think it was a beaver."

The neighbor answered, "We don't have any beavers around this area. It was probably a ground hog. In fact, I just saw a ground hog going to church this morning."

The young son chimed in, "How did you know it was going to church?"

Or this one?

One day a husband came home and saw a lot of flowers and plants all over the house.

The husband asked his wife, "Where did you get all these flowers?"

His wife replied, "I just did what you told me to do."

The husband inquired, "What do you mean you did what I told you to do?"

The wife said, "You said when I went to visit my friend, Mary, at the hospital, that I should be sure and take her flowers. So, I took them!"

Here is another good one.

Tony walked in to Joe's Barber Shop for his regular haircut. As he snips away, Joe asks, "What's up?"

Tony says, "We're taking a vacation to Rome."

"Rome?" Joe says, "Why would you want to go there? It's a crowded dirty city full of Italians! You'd be crazy to go to Rome! So how ya getting there?"

"We're taking TWA," Tony replies.

"TWA?!" yells Joe. "They're a terrible airline. The planes are old, their flight attendants are ugly, and they're always late! So where you staying in Rome?"

Tony says, "We'll be at the Downtown International Marriot."

"That dump?!" says Joe. That's the worst hotel in the city! The rooms are small, the service is surly and slow, and they're overpriced! So whatcha doing when you get there?"

Tony replies, "We're going to go see the Vatican and hope to see the Pope."

"Ha! That's rich!" laughs Joe. "You and a million other people trying to see him. He'll look the size of an ant. Boy, good luck on *this* trip. You're going to need it!"

A month later, Tony comes in for his regular haircut. Joe says, "Well, how did that trip to Rome turn out? Betcha TWA gave you the worst flight of your life!"

"No, quite the opposite." explained Tony. "Not only were we on time and in one of their brand new planes, but it was full, so they bumped us up to first class. The food and drinks were wonderful and we had a beautiful young flight attendant who waited on us hand and foot!"

"Hmmmm," Joe says, "well, I bet the hotel was just like I described."

"Nope, just the opposite!" said Tony. "They'd just finished a $25 million remodel. It's the finest hotel in Rome now. They were overbooked, so they apologized and gave us the presidential suite for no extra charge!"

"Well," mumbles Joe, "I *know* you didn't get to see the Pope!"

"Actually, we were quite lucky. As we toured the Vatican, a Swiss guard tapped me on the shoulder and explained the Pope likes to personally meet some of the visitors, and if I'd be so kind as to step into this private room and wait, the Pope would personally greet us.

Sure enough, after five minutes the Pope walked through the door and shook my hand. I knelt down as he spoke a few words to me."

Impressed, Joe asks, "Tell me, please! What'd he say?"

"Oh, not much really," Tony replies, just, "Where'd you get that awful haircut!"

Or did you hear this one about two friends that were at their other friend Joe's funeral?

The first friend said, "Boy, doesn't Joe look good?"

The second friend said, "Well, he should. He just came from the hospital!"

This is funny, but unfortunately, all too true. We've been in the hospital at different times and have heard that one of the patients had passed away. How many famous people have we all heard about (on the news) that pass away while in the hospital? How many people do we personally know that have passed away while in a hospital?

If one were to open a funeral parlor, it would be a smart idea to put it right next to a hospital. Who knows what time and costs it might save?

These oldies but goodies will make you laugh!

Videos:

No Time for Sergeants with Andy Griffith

Anything with Yakov Smirnoff. And if you are in Branson, Missouri, be sure you go to see his show!

Almost anything with Red Skelton. My sister and her husband went to see one of his live shows. He was on stage performing for over two hours and then did another half-hour encore. Afterwards he asked the audience if they realized that they sat for over two and a half hours and did not hear one swear word or any dirty jokes. He got a standing ovation for that!

Bob Hope keeps it clean, too. When comedians keep it clean, they rarely offend anyone.

Victor Borges is not only hilarious but a fantastic piano player. He usually only plays really well near the end of the videos.

Cassette tapes (probably available on CD):

Burns and Allen (George Burns and Gracie Allen)

Jack Benny

Fibber McGee and Molly

These may be old, but they will really tickle your funny bone—for a good, hard, belly laugh!

There are many more out there to be had. I've only listed the ones we have that are still very funny after seeing or hearing them over and over.

Any day with Laughter is a good day

---

[1] "Longevity" December 1988 "Laughter is Good Medicine" by Robert Brody

Chapter Nine

HERE WE GO AGAIN!

I didn't expect that Chuck and I would have another episode of *Proof is in the Pudding* to help convince us that conventional medicine had it all wrong. Chuck would again be the guinea pig for another chapter in this book!

On Friday October 7, 2011, we were just leaving South Bend, Ind. after a week's stay in Amish country. Chuck didn't feel too well so I drove home to Michigan. When we got home, he said he needed to lie down and would help unload the car later. There wasn't anything too heavy, so I did it so that he could rest. Later in the evening he still felt bad and complained of a severe stomach ache. When I asked if he wanted to go to the emergency room at the hospital, he said no.

At about 3:00 a.m., he said I could drive him to St. Joseph Mercy Hospital in Ypsilanti, Michigan or call 911. We got dressed and I drove. The fog was very thick and we could only see a few feet in front of the car, so the trip was very slow.

At the hospital, Chuck was given a small dose of morphine to ease his pain. The doctors and nurses checked his vitals and determined he was experiencing atrial fibrillation (A-fib—very fast heart rate), an infection, pancreatitis, and jaundice. By 4:30 a.m. he was taken to the Intensive Care Unit (ICU).

He was hooked up to heart monitors, an IV of saline solution, medication to slow his heart rate, and nutrients. The doctors couldn't put a scope down his throat to see what was wrong in the stomach and pancreas until his heart rate was lowered.

At 2:00 a.m. Sunday morning, a doctor put a couple of small tubes in Chuck's neck. He was taken for an X-ray, but returned when staff found that the tubes were too long, so the doctor came back and shortened them.

About 10:00 a.m. Sunday, the doctors said the medication was not slowing his heart rate, which was up to over 200 beats per minute and was instead only lowering his blood pressure. His blood pressure was getting very low. They needed my permission to give him a shock treatment to force the heart rhythm back to normal. If it wasn't done within forty-eight hours, he could have a stroke or heart attack. Of course, I gave my permission.

Chuck was sedated and taken to a surgical area where he was given the shock treatment

About 2:00 p.m. he was sedated again and taken to have the scope put down his throat. They found an eight millimeter gall stone, lots of "sledge," puss, and several small stones, which they were able to remove through the scope. The large stone was blocking the gall bladder from doing its job, causing the infection and other matter to back into his liver and pancreas. They also enlarged the opening in the gall bladder to pass any further stones. In spite of all these procedures, the doctors recommended he have his gall bladder removed.

One of the doctors wanted to do the operation while he was still in the hospital. I said I'd like to wait until he had recovered some and was in better health. Dr. David M. Winston agreed with me. We liked this doctor the best, he was friendly and a good sense of humor.

While Chuck's sedatives were wearing off he had a few words to say to me, "Did you do this to me on purpose!" And, "Go get the nurse and let's get out of here, I need to go to the hospital." I didn't do what I suggested you do in an earlier chapter, "Don't leave home without them."

Since my dear hubby was somewhat out of the woods on Tuesday, I finally went home to bathe (so the hospital wouldn't have to fumigate the room) and especially to get the vitamins and minerals that he needed. Even if we had thought to grab the vitamin C and coral calcium, I certainly could not have known he would need the iodine.

Chuck's heart rate was still quite high, varying between 171 and 153 beats per minute. It should be under 100. Remember, Chuck had received the shock treatment three days prior on Saturday at 10:00 a.m. to regulate his heart rate.

On the following Tuesday evening after returning from home, I gave him the first two drops of Iosol (food-grade Iodine) to regulate his pulse and put two packages of Emergen-C in his supper juice for his liver (bilirubin level) and blood pressure. All this was two-and-a-half days after the shock treatment to regulate his pulse.

Chuck continued to take two drops of iodine and two packages of Emergen-C with each meal. I also gave him two Ester-C tablets, two Coral Calcium pills, and two Resveratrol Plus tablets a couple times a day. This was all done, of course, without anyone at the hospital's knowledge!

On Wednesday (the following morning):

a.m. : Pulse 103 Blood pressure 141/98 Billa-rubin (liver) 15 (normal should be between 1 and 2)
p.m.: Pulse 77 Blood Pressure 128/58 Liver 11

Thursday: (moved out of the ICU)

a.m.: Pulse 68 Blood Pressure 135/59 Liver 8.2
p.m.: Pulse 70 n/a Liver n/a Only check blood a.m.

Friday:

a.m.: Pulse 65 Blood pressure 134/69 Liver 6.6

Doctor David M. Winston said to Chuck, "You're making amazing progress—probably because your wife is here!" To me he said, "You make a great nurse!" Prophetic words, because he had no idea of what Chuck was getting each day in iodine, vitamins, and minerals.

p.m.: Pulse 68 Blood pressure 128/62

Saturday:

a.m.: Pulse 69 Blood pressure 143/70 Liver 6.2
p.m.: Pulse 68 Blood pressure 131/67

Sunday:

a.m.: Pulse 72 Blood pressure 138/68 Liver 5.4

He was sent home before lunch on Sunday. He was supposed to have "Home Care" for a month or longer, if needed. Also, he was instructed to make an appointment with our regular doctor for the following Tuesday.

Under "Medications" on the "Discharge Instructions" given to Chuck when he was released from the hospital, Chuck was instructed to take were:

Multivitamin (Vitamin B Complex (Foltx)
Multivitamin with minerals (Vitafol Therapeutic Multiple Vitamins and minerals oral tablet)
Omega-3, polyunsaturated fatty acids (Fish Oil-oral capsule)
Ascorbic acid (vitamin C)
Ubiquinone (Co-Q10)
Zinc chloride
Thyroid desiccated (Armoir Thyroid)
Aspirin, 81 mg
Metoprolol (metoprolol 50 mg oral tablet)

At first I thought it unusual that the Hospital would list vitamins under "Medications." These were the vitamins that he was already taking, that he could remember, when he was in pain and went into the hospital in the first place. Then it hit me—could it possibly be another attempt to make vitamins "prescription only" in the future? When this thought came to me, then it did make sense to list vitamins under "Medications"!

We went to a Tuesday appointment at our regular doctor; the staff checked all his vitals and took some blood samples. They said they would call us on Wednesday if there was anything negative and if he needed to come in. We received no call. The doctor's office did call on Thursday and wants Chuck to come in next week, for a follow-up blood test to see if everything is still improving as well as it was in the hospital by the "professional" staff. This "unprofessional" is still giving Chuck the Iosol, but only one drop twice a day and the vitamin C, however, slightly less. (The older we get the more vitamin C we need for good health.)

Chuck has started taking milk thistle and peppermint (mint sugar free candies and mint tea) which is recommended for gall bladder problems in a few of the health books we have by alternative doctors.

So, unfortunately, Chuck had to go through all of this and be once again close to "checking out." But now we personally know that Iosol (iodine) really does lower the heart rate and does so, rather quickly. We know that vitamin C is an additional aid, especially for bilirubin levels and pancreatic function.

This experience provides more proof that natural, God-given cures do work and that doctors need to be taught about vitamins, minerals, and herbs in their extensive schooling so that they can really help people! But vitamins should not be "prescription only!" Buying what vitamins we want and when we want them is just fine—the way it is now.

I cannot say enough on how important it is to resist the power that the pharmaceutical companies, the FDA, the AMA, and our government have over our very lives! Things need to change or our health is at stake; more and more deaths will continue to occur from the drugs that "big pharma" invents and pushes on us (through doctors and advertising). Their "licensed to kill" has continued far too long!

The next chapter highlights only a portion of how much control our government now has over us; more and more control is continuing to be added and is taking away more and more of our freedoms.

Chapter Ten

GOVERNMENT *OF* THE PEOPLE?

Our country was founded on the principle of "government of the people, by the people, and for the people" but now it seems like government "controls" the people.

Our bodies are mostly made up of water. So, drinking good quality water is of the utmost importance. The municipal water in our cities is full of toxins—most is supplemented with fluoride and chlorine among other chemicals. Fluoride was originally a waste substance left over from the aluminum industry that manufacturers didn't know how to get rid of. Aluminum is a substance that has been found in the brains of victims of Alzheimer's disease. Fluoride can be tied to discolored teeth, brain damage, arthritis, muscle disorders, infertility, and more.

The aluminum companies sure get rid of it now with most all cities in the good ole U.S. of A. adding fluoride (and chlorine) to all the water that we are supposed to bathe in, wash cloths in, water our gardens with, and, heaven forbid, *drink*!

There are a few cities in the United States that have ceased adding fluoride to their water by mandates of city government. Fairbanks, Alaska; Mount Clemens, Michigan; Marcellus, Michigan; and Independence, Virginia were the only ones at the time this book was written.[1] These are just individual cities. If you don't live in one of these cities, adding a drop or two of Iosol (iodine) will help mitigate the effects of these chemicals. Buying spring or distilled water or one of the pitcher filters now available is another solution. European countries that used to add fluoride to their water no longer add this poisonous substance. Are their governments much wiser than the US government?

Fortunately Chuck and I live in the country and have well water. We also purchase Absopure water for drinking.

Our Government controls are getting even worse! One of the schools in Alabama does not allow the children to bring any kind of drinks from home. The only drinks they are allowed is, that's right, city water—one of the worst, most unhealthy substances you can put into your body!

If you think you have freedom of choice, think again! And watch the news broadcasts. For instance,

in the state of Pennsylvania, teachers are trying to decide how to limit what and how many treats the children will be allowed to share with the other students. The state of New York had banned some desserts, such as cupcakes, to share with the class, in at least one of their school systems. In Arizona, no child's lunch can contain items made with sugar or white flour. And in Chicago, believe it or not, no lunches may be brought from home. The Chicago school district claims that its cafeteria food is more nutritional and better quality than any lunch a parent can make. The list goes on. Fast foods are not allowed in some schools. It is well-known that sugar, white flour, pop, and most fast foods are not on the top of the list of a healthy diet.

Why have parents lost the control of what their children are allowed to eat? Wouldn't classes teaching nutrition be more healthful than having the government control what children can or cannot put in their mouths? The children would probably love to bring their newly-learned information on nutrition home to their parents. I'm sure the parents would love to hear all their children have to say. This could make for some very good and enjoyable conversations at the dinner table.

Teachers are supposed to be for teaching, not for snooping through a student's lunch or forbidding them to bring a lunch from home at all. Parents are supposed to be the ones deciding what is best for their own children! School officials in Massachusetts took the American flag away from a seventh-grade student.

Our country is getting closer and closer to socialism almost every day and it's scary! If a child is considered too obese, he or she can be taken away from his or her parents and put into a foster home.

One of these cases is a twelve-year-old child who weighed a few hundred pounds. She was taken from her parents and put into a foster care house. (A house is not "home.") Certainly this much weight is not a good thing for her physical health, but what is being taking away from her family and being placed with strangers, doing to her emotional and mental health?

The law now requires health care providers to report children they think to be in danger from any abuse, neglect, or any circumstance that could mean "failure to thrive." This is about as open to interpretation as it can get. There are children that have been taken from parents for being *victims* of spanking! What's happened to the biblical saying, "spare the rod and spoil the child"? Want to see a future juvenile delinquent? Then just look at a child that is not disciplined!

In the interest of keeping families together *and* healthy, why not offer classes on diet, nutrition, and health to both the parents and the children?

This could do them both good and they would remain a family! Where are the hearts and brains of our legal system?

Our freedoms and choices are being taking away from us at almost every turn, all under the guise of the government knowing what is best for us more than we do! Where does this government control end? The government wants to control the big things as well as the little things in our lives.

The government is now ordering more and more companies to reduce the salt in their products. This is probably a good thing, because most of the salt they use is chemically processed. The salt we should use is a natural sea salt. Again, read the Labels. A good sea salt needs to be stirred or shaken up every so often to keep it from hardening into a solid lump.

The government also requires salt manufacturers to add Iodine. This would be good if it were real sea salt and if it weren't for the fluoride and chlorine that is added to cities' water supplies. (People use water in much of their cooking.) These chemicals and processed salt cancels out the good effects of the iodine.

Restricting peoples' salt consumption could even be dangerous! Very few people are sensitive to sodium. Restricting salt in summer months could really be dangerous when heat exhaustion, fainting, and stroke are all a greater risk.

Remember when my husband spent nine days in the hospital because of a statin drug (simvastatin) and again more recently another eight days. Both times was given an IV saline solution to flush his body. Saline solutions are often given to hospital patients. Saline solution is made with *salt*! If salt were really so bad for us, why do hospitals load our bodies with saline solutions? So somewhere someone knows that salt has medicinal benefits!

There are some doctors that have become aware that their patients who use little salt are the patients with high blood pressure.[2] A few have even been noticing that the blood pressure begins to decline when they use more salt. So who came up with the idea that salt is bad for us? And why did we all fall for it?

Less than ten percent of people *may* be sensitive to sodium. A fairly new study shows that the individuals who ate less salt are more likely to die from heart diseases than those who do not restrict their salt intake. [3] This doesn't mean, however, to make your food look like it has been "snow" covered!

We put out a block of salt near our woods (we live in the country) and the deer, especially, flock to it. The ground around the salt block is loaded with deer hoof prints. Animals are usually smart and know what is and isn't good for them. You can't convince animals that salt is bad for them—government or no government!

Speaking of animals being smart about what to eat and what not to eat, deer and fowl will not eat soy beans. And yet soy is touted as a health food. We are offered soy burgers, soy cereal, soy this, and soy that! Deer will eat your tulip bulbs, but not your daffodil bulbs—the daffodil bulbs are poisonous to them. Animals have a sixth sense, so maybe we should take a lesson from them. They seem to know a lot more than we do about what is good for us and what isn't!

People have drunk raw milk for thousands of years. It contains good bacteria and is healthier than pasteurized milk, which contains bad bacteria. In fact, pasteurized milk can be downright dangerous. There were more than several hundred cases of food poisoning and deaths due to pasteurized milk a while back.

My in-laws used to drink milk that came straight from their cow. It went from the cow, into a bucket, and then to their glasses. Their parents, and ancestors, did the same. If raw milk were so dangerous, they should be dead. And if they were dead, we wouldn't even be here, and neither would you!

My in-laws gave us what most people call a "pie safe" that was made by my husband's grandfather. When I called it a "pie safe" my mother-in-law corrected me. She informed me that it was a "milk safe." She said we never had very many pies to put in it, but we had milk to put in it every single day. The "milk safe" was used to keep the flies away from the milk.

They probably put a silver spoon in the milk too. Some of you may be old enough to recall your grandmother used to put a silver spoon in the bucket of raw milk to keep it from spoiling too fast. Remember from chapter seven on colloidal silver about its ability to kill all the bad microorganisms.

The US Department of Agriculture's data shows that the consumers of pasteurized/homogenized milk are twenty-nine times more likely to get sick than those who drink raw milk! If you can find raw milk, by all means buy it. The government now also has laws about not selling raw milk!

The following excerpt is copied from a report [4] by William Douglas, MD. He suggested making copies to give to your friends especially if they are in the military. I'll take his advice because I'm considering anyone that reads this book a friend.

Soldiers forced to receive untested shots

Whether or not you support the war in Iraq, I certainly hope you support the men and women who are putting their lives on the line every single day. Sometimes, though, I can't help but wonder which side of the War in Iraq Washington DC is actually on—especially when they start using our troops as human guinea pigs.

The latest scandal involves a substance that was never clinically tested and that every single soldier is required to have jabbed into his arm. The soldiers are finally catching wind of the side effects of this untested substance (heart disease, kidney failure, and multiple sclerosis, for example), and they're none too happy about it. In fact, there's a growing rebellion among the troops—even officers—to this unethical abuse of power. You can hardly blame them. This isn't exactly what they signed up for. [5]

Of course, the strong arm of the military has a thing or two to say about such open acts of rebellion. I'll say more on that a little later. First, you need to know a little about this mandatory shot called the anthrax vaccine.

Gulf War Syndrome all over again

Mandatory shots are nothing new. I remember getting shots (without my permission, though it never would have occurred to me to refuse them. What does an 18-year-old sailor know?), but in 1945 there weren't many of them, and they were relatively innocuous.

So the concept wasn't new in 1991, when the massive injection of unproved vaccines gained momentum in the first Gulf War. Anthrax and other vaccines (many of them of questionable use and safety) were forced on the troops under King George the first. The risk level of severe illness, lifetime disability, and even death was something no one counted on and plenty would like to sweep under the rug.

I know it's been a while since the "Gulf War Syndrome" was on the tips of every one's tongues. So in case you're a bit rusty on the details, allow me to polish your memory a bit.

When our Desert Storm vets came home, many brought more than just nightmares with them. Symptoms such as chronic fatigue, loss of muscle control, headaches, shortness of breath, and even diabetes became so common that they were all lumped under on heading: Gulf War Syndrome (GWS).

Plenty of studies have been done over the years, and out of the potential causes, one cause stands out like a sore thumb: side effects from the anthrax vaccine. And for those who would point a finger at chemical weapons or parasitic diseases, try this on for size: Even troops that were never deployed overseas have developed GWS. Yes, the common enemy—both of the soldiers on the war front and on the home front—was from our own government: again, the mandatory anthrax vaccine.

Did you know that the FDA approved the vaccine even though it never went through a single, large-scale, clinical trial?

Of all the nations involved in actual combat, the two with the highest rates of excess illness were the United States and the Great Britain—the two nations with the highest reported uses of pesticides and the anthrax vaccine. France, on the other hand, didn't use the anthrax vaccine and had the lowest rates of illness. Coincidence? I don't think so.

Now, more than a decade later, King George II is in power, and the deadly charade continues in the Gulf War II.

The military takes aim at its own troops

In 2008, the soldiers who received the vaccine are facing the same risks as those who went before them. According to the General accounting Office (GAO), they're anticipating that at least one to two percent of those who get the shot could experience what they're calling "adverse events"—in plain English, this means side effects that can lead to disability or death. Two percent might not sound like much to you—but that's two percent of 2.2 million servicemen and women who have received the mandatory shot. That's over 22,000 soldiers that they expect to develop a disability or die from a shot that the FDA says is "safe and effective."

Isn't it amazing that we have to depend on the General Accounting Office to find the truth? Where is Bethesda Naval Hospital? Walter Reed Army Medical Center? The Department of Health and Human Services? The FDA? The CDC? The Ministry of Truth and Human Virtue (a little humor)? They are all about as responsive as those stone statues on Easter Island—looking to the sea and revealing nothing.

The anthrax vaccine is called BioThrax, and it's made by a company called Emergent Biosolutions (previously BioPort). The Pentagon asserts that it is safe, but the company's own insurance company isn't so sure. In fact, the Evanston Insurance company actually sued BioPort, "alleging 'material misrepresentations' by the pharmaceutical company about 'incidents, conditions, circumstances, defects, or suspected defects' in the vaccine." In the old days, we called this *fraud* and it got you ten years in the slammer. Now such criminal behavior is rewarded with bigger and better contracts.

According to WorldNetDaily, "The military suspended the use of the anthrax vaccine in October 2004 in response to a court order revealing concerns over the process through which it was approved for use on the military, but that order expired in October 2006 and the mandatory shots were resumed within a few months."

It just . . . *expired*? Not one single of Congress's one hundred senators said, "Wait a minute! What have you done to prove the soldiers and many scientists wrong?" Well, the answer (had the question been raised) would have been that they had done nothing. The court order just expired after two years of no action. The con artists known as your elected public servants know that the average voter can't remember what happened two weeks ago let alone two *years* ago.

Couldn't they have at least reemployed the ban and forced a full investigation? Of course they could have, but instead they've deserted your children, your spouse, your sweetheart, your grandchildren—just as the military has done.

Believe it or not, the government actually admits that the vaccine could possibly have killed as many as twenty-one soldiers. That they admit it has killed *any* is pretty darn surprising—especially since they're standing by their claim that it's "safe and effective." But just imagine how many deaths they're *not* admitting to. I've come across plenty of credible sources that indicate the number is much higher, but because it's not "proven" and because the government hasn't admitted to it (And why would they?), the numbers cannot be published.

I realize this might sound a bit callous, but dying might be considered the easy way out. Those who survive are forced to live with the painful debilitating side effects that often affects them for the rest of their lives. Thousands have suffered from nervous system disorders skin disorders, and bone disorders. And a few have even developed heart problems, seizures, diabetes, multiple sclerosis, inflammatory arthritis, and even lesions on the brain.

Trying to save face, the GAO's best explanation is that "some of these events may occur coincidentally following immunization, while others may truly be caused by the immunization." Bull. These men and women were all cleared and certified in good health on entering the military. How does an eighteen-year-old come down with diabetes, heart disease, or multiple sclerosis coincidentally?

So what's a soldier to do? A soldier's body is not his own

These stats aren't exactly a secret anymore and the troops aren't too thrilled. Some of them have seen Gulf War Syndrome first-hand and know of its connection to the anthrax vaccine. Yet they have no choice but to watch as the needle gets jabbed into their arm and the deadly "juice" slowly gets injected into their blood stream with the push of a thumb. Their only "acceptable" course of action is to cross their fingers or pray to whoever they think they're going to meet if they become a statistic.

It's one thing to die for your country, but dying for a pharmaceutical company? It's not exactly what our soldiers signed up for. The story of Leif

Hamre illustrates the vice these soldiers are finding themselves in.

Private Leif Hamre is a special sort of private, and not exactly what the military wants at that level (or any level for that matter). He thinks for himself and speaks out when others dare not. Yes, I know the military is not a democracy. You have to take orders from those above you. You are a killing machine, not a "peace force," which is an oxymoron, anyway. But when you insult the intelligence of your men and rob them of the right to protect themselves against an obvious enemy—which the anthrax vaccine has been proven to be—you create a deep resentment, along with a quiet rebellion and a fall in morale.

When Private Hamre discovered that the vaccine hadn't been properly stored, he refused to receive it. The military's reaction was predictable. According to WorldNetDaily, "Hamre was awarded with eighteen-hour work days, he was taken off missions, and his pay scale was lowered."

In an open letter to friends and family members, he said, "The tactics they have used to coerce me into taking the [anthrax] shot that is unregulated, are unscrupulous and downright un-American."

Having ten years in the military (two separate enlistments), I will say that Lief made a serious error here. He insulted the military brass and for that he will be severely punished. The fact that he is telling the truth is irrelevant. As I iterated above, the military is a killing machine and blind obedience is essential for success.

The fact that he enlisted voluntarily weakens his case. He was badly advised (if he was advised at all) before making a decision to "fight for democracy and freedom" in a country (Iraq) that doesn't care about either. They care about Islam—democracy and freedom are not in their lexicon. Now he has two enemies: Islamic fundamentalists *and* the American military. Who should he pray to now?

Your Part in this Story

If all of this isn't enough to get you up in arms, perhaps this next bit of information will: you could be next. At any given time, the government could mandate that *you* get this shot as well. Dr. Meryl Nass, a board-certified internist who is opposed to the anthrax vaccine, says that it is "legally and technically possible" that all Americans will be forced to take the vaccine.

She offered a possible scenario: if a handful of people were to be exposed in an office building in Los Angeles, for example, the government could issue an order for vaccination for everybody in the building, maybe even everybody in Los Angeles. That's what people now are facing.

So that raises the question: what can be done?

Well, as Sir Francis Bacon said, "Knowledge is power." Read more about it. Talk to people about it. By all means, if you know someone who is in the military, share this article with them. Point them to a few informative websites, like Dr. Nass's site: www. anthraxvaccine.org. In fact, Dr. Nass is so passionate about this cause that she's offering to do a *free* video conference with servicemen. Visit her website to find out the details.

There is help out there, but the initial resistance and leadership comes from non-scientists—Americans with common sense who may or may not have a degree in science. Lyme disease, for example, was not discovered by a scientist but by a Connecticut housewife from Lyme, Connecticut. A "real" scientist then isolated the organism. She deserves the credit for thinking outside the medical box and pointing the scientists in the right direction. She should have been awarded with a Nobel Prize.

One person leading the way in the anthrax fight is investigative journalist Gary Matsumoto. His book, *Vaccine-A*, clearly connects the anthrax vaccine to Gulf War Syndrome. Some of the cases he describes are gruesome, even to a doctor. You owe it to yourself, your family, and your much-abused country to read it.

Marguerite Armisted is from an organization called Protecting Our Guardians, an ironically appropriate title for citizens trying to protect our soldiers from the excesses of military medicine. "In this military program, we have a product that has led to numerous fatalities, numerous adverse reactions, and yet soldiers are told they won't be deployable if they don't take this," she said. The intended victim should have responded, "Then don't deploy me." Armisted went on to say, "This really is like Russian roulette. Put three bullets in, spin the chamber and take your shot."

And remember: You may be next.

Copied from "The Best of the Douglass Report" by Dr. William Campbell Douglass, II, M.D. Volume VII Used by Permission

Rates of autism and learning-disabled children have soared since our children started getting vaccinated. Fifty years ago there was only one child in 2,000[6] that were considered autistic. In 2008[7], in the US Department of Health and Human Services survey, it was one in eighty eight! There are now more than two-and-a-half-million autistic children in the United States. Since the mass vaccination of children began in 1990, the rise in autism has continued to explode dramatically! The number of vaccinations for mumps, measles, and chicken pox forced upon our children has sky rocketed in the last twenty-five years.

Are these diseases worse than learning disabilities and autism? Yet the drug companies are free and clear of any liabilities. A law (Public Law 99-660, the National Childhood Vaccine Injury Act) passed in 1986 signed by a reluctant President, Ronald Reagan, reads, "No vaccine manufacturer shall be liable in a civil action for damages arising from a vaccine-related injury or death!"

This chapter is a small illustration of how our current government is beginning more and more to control us in the good ole' U.S.A.

Is America the "land of the free" or is it becoming "The land of the government and the land of the pharmaceutical companies"?

We need to do something about it! And if not now, when? Our health and even our lives are at stake!

We've come to the conclusion
That Drugs are just a delusion—
And should be an exclusion
That we will be refusin'
They're a dangerous intrusion!
If you think you may be Ill
Then you better take a pill
If you think you will be sick
Then you better take it quick!
And when it's from big pharma
It sure can do you harm-a
It's the little pill to kill
From the big pharmaceutical

If you think the preceding was scary enough regarding our government and the powers of the organizations such as the FDA, just read the next few pages written by Garret W. Wood, President of Advanced Bionutritionals! (Used with his permission, as long as it is copied verbatim).[8]

Read, and then take the action he recommends or the supplements that you are now taking could become unavailable and your health (and even your life) could be at risk!

Advanced Bionutritionals

P.O. Box 8051—Norcross, GA 30091-8051-1-800-791-3395

Dear friend,

This is the most serious message I've ever had to write to you.

Why? Because the FDA has issued new rules that, if enacted, will enable them to ban many of the supplements you are now taking.

Think I'm exaggerating? /then please listen to the full story . . .

Back in the early 1990s, the FDA tried to make many supplements illegal. Consumers were so alarmed by the FDA's bullying that they staged a massive revolt. The result was that Congress passed the Dietary Supplement Health and Education Act (DSHEA). That law protected supplements from FDA unless the FDA could prove a supplement wasn't safe.

There was, however, a loophole in the 1994 law. The FDA was given the authority to regulate new ingredients introduced after October 15, 1994.

So what happened? Nothing at first. For 17 years, the dietary supplement industry has enjoyed tremendous innovations. These innovations have allowed us to extract and concentrate the most effective natural ingredients. As a result, millions of consumers have benefited. They've protected their hearts and arteries . . . found relief from their joint pain . . . boosted their memory . . . and more.

And during this time, supplements have enjoyed a remarkable safety record. Statistics show that supplements are safer than prescription drugs, cosmetics, medical devices, and even food!

According to the Poison Control Centers, there were zero deaths due to supplements in 2008. In 2009, there was one.

Meanwhile, pathogens like E coli in food kill at least 2,000 people each year. Acetaminophen in drugs like Tylenol kills 450 people every year. And more powerful prescription drugs kill many more. Even the FDA now says Vioxx likely killed over 26,000 people before they finally took it off the market!

Supplements the FDA Wants to Ban

But now the FDA wants to act like the last 17 years never happened. The agency has drafted a proposal to regulate what it calls New Dietary Ingredients. If this proposal is implemented, some of the most effective nutrients you take will be pulled from the market. Nutrients like resveratrol—ubiquinol CoQ10—bacopa—strontium—and more.

But that's not all. Under these guidelines, and FDA can define almost *anything* as a "new" dietary ingredient. For example:

- If a supplement includes more of an ingredient than was used 17 years ago—even something like vitamin C—it's "new".
- If an ingredient uses a different extraction process—like baking or fermentation—it's "new".
- If a supplement uses an ingredient at a different "life stage"—such as using ripe rather than non-ripe apples—it's "new".
- If a supplement duplicates an ingredient in a laboratory rather than extracting it from the food—even though it's chemically identical—it's "new".
- And if a probiotic formula includes a strain of bacteria that wasn't found in yogurt 17 years ago, it's "new".

So what would happen to all these "new" ingredients? The manufacturers would have to take them off the market until they could *prove* the ingredients have been safely used for 17 years!

Why It's Nearly Impossible to Comply

What kind of proof is the FDA demanding? According to the guidelines, many companies would have to conduct animal studies using a dosage that's *1,000 times* the typical dose.

I'm not kidding you. It's right there in black and white on the FDA's website. The FDA wants vitamin makers to do studies for a full year, at 1,000 times the typical dose.

So a fish oil manufacturer would have to conduct a one-year study where animals are force-fed the human equivalent of 240,000 milligrams of fish oil each and every day! This outlandish dose would injure the animals and give the FDA an excuse to outlaw the product.

But wait, it gets even better. If one fish-oil manufacturer performs such a study and it passes, it doesn't mean the other fish-oil makers can use the same data. No sir. They are still required to go out and do their own studies before they're allowed to sell their product.

And these studies are very expensive. A study like the one above typically costs about $100,000—$200,000 to perform. Multiply that by several ingredients in several products, and you get an idea of the costs.

Say a company carries 6 products containing 6 ingredients each. It would cost between $3.6 and $7.2 million in studies before that company could even offer the products for sale. For a larger company offering 50 products or more, the costs would be astronomical.

Few supplement makers will be able to afford these studies, and many will be put out of business. And the ones that remain would still be at the mercy of the FDA's whim. That's because there are no requirements for the FDA to approve anything. They can approve or reject anything they want. And in the past, they have rejected the majority of ingredients submitted to them.

That means most of the nutrients you buy today will be pulled from the market and never return. Those that do return will be a lot more expensive—or may only be available as prescription drugs!

A Blatant Abuse of Power

This is a blatant abuse of power. What the FDA is doing here is performing an end-run around the existing law. According to the law, the FDA has to prove a dietary supplement is unsafe for it to be taken off the market. These new guidelines turn that on its head. They are clearly not what Congress intended.

Fortunately, these FDA guidelines have not yet been finalized. All federal agencies are required to give the pubic an opportunity to comment on a draft before it is made final. In this case, the FDA has given interested parties until December 1st to comment on the draft. That means there's a small window of opportunity for you to voice your disapproval.

Frankly, I wouldn't bother commenting to the FDA. The process is cumbersome, and those unelected bureaucrats don't care what you think anyway.

What You Can Do

The best way to defeat these new rules is to talk to the people you do elect—your congressman and your two U.S. senators. They have the power to reign in the FDA—and they have done so in the past when enough voters complained.

Back in the 1970's, the FDA tried to require "warning labels" on vitamins. Angry voters called and wrote letters, and Congress responded with the Proxmire Amendments which limited the FDA's power.

Then in the 1990s, the FDA went on the warpath again. When voters complained, Congress passed the Dietary Health Supplement Education Act, which once again limited the FDA's power.

But like a monster killed in a horror movie, the FDA keeps coming back. And so once again, it's time for us to step up and call the folks who rely on our votes.

Here's what you need to do:

Go to

www.usa.gov/Contact/Elected.shtml.

That web address is case sensitive. So type it exactly as it appears. On the website, look up the phone numbers of your U.S. Senators and your Representative (congressman). Then give them a call.

Don't be shy and don't worry. No one is going to bite you, no one is going to argue with you, and no one is going to quiz you to see how well you know the issues. The job of the staffers who answer is to listen politely and to relay what you say to their boss. So please do call. And please be polite and respectful of the staffers' time.

Here are some talking points to use when you call:

* Hello, my name is [name] and I am a constituent of [name of Senator or Representative].
* I am concerned about the new FDA draft guidance on dietary supplements and new dietary ingredients.

* [Feel free to tell them about the supplements you take and/or the benefits you get from those supplements. Then feel free to make as many of the following points as you like:]

1. Supplements have an unrivaled safety record. Statistics show they're safer than drugs, safer than medical devices, safer than cosmetics, and even safer than food.

2. The FDA cannot define New Dietary Ingredients so broadly. According to these guidelines, almost everything is a New Dietary Ingredient. This will strangle innovation and deprive consumers of the supplements they depend on for their health.

3. The FDA did nothing about new dietary ingredients for 17 years. Now they want to wipe out 17 years' worth of innovation and 17 years' worth of benefits to the consumer.

4. When the Dietary Health Supplement Education Act was passed, Congress intended a simple notification process for new dietary ingredients. The FDA is turning this into a pre-approval scheme, which goes against the intent of the law.

5. The FDA already has ample regulatory authority to take action against a product if it's unsafe. They don't need to have this pre-approval power, too.

6. These could be disastrous to public health. At a time when preventative measures are even more important to health care costs, the FDA is limiting access to preventative health care.

7. The cost of complying with these guidelines would be astronomical. Experts estimate that the studies required would cost between $100,000 and $200,000 per ingredient notification. That adds up to millions of dollars per supplement company. Smaller companies would not be able to afford this and would go out of business.

   The economy is already hurting and we have high unemployment. Experts estimate that this could cost the economy tens of billions of dollars and result in the loss of tens of thousands of jobs.

8. The government's resources are already stretched. We have record budget deficits and record debt. Why enact more regulations when there are no safety issues here?

* I request that Congress direct the FDA to carefully review their draft guidance. If they do not amend their guidance to reflect my concerns, I request that Congress call hearings at the end of the review process. I also call on Congress to write legislation that would "grandfather" all supplements currently on the market.
* Thank you for your time.

After the phone call, send a letter to your senators and reps making the same points. Make sure your letter is in your own words (form letters tend not to work as well). You can find the e-mail and physical addresses at the same website, www.usa.gov/Contact/Elected.shtml. Don't forget that link is case sensitive.

Then send the same letter to President Obama. (His address and phone number are on the website, too.)

Please, please, please don't make the mistake of thinking that the FDA won't take your supplements away. Similar regulations were passed in other countries, and the result was disastrous. Many supplements were taken off the market forever. In some instances, the entire supplement industry was decimated. Don't let that happen here.

Take action now! You only have a small window of opportunity to make your voice heard. Get started by going to www.usa.gov/Contact/Elected.shtml.

Sincerely,

Garret W. Wood
President, Advanced Bionutritionals

The following article is from Dr. Robert Jay Rowen's *Second Opinion* newsletter, Vol. XX11, No. 4, April 2012. It is and copied as written with permission granted.[9]

Global Attacks on Alternative Medicine Escalate

You've read in these pages about the various attacks our government has attempted against alternative medicine. Whether it's raids on doctors' offices and whole-food markets or new laws set up to destroy us, our government is actively seeking to destroy your medical freedom. In recent months, those attacks have escalated. But they're not just here in the U.S. It's a global phenomenon.

For instance, in Europe, recent laws have regulated many supplements as drugs. And it's forced many of them off the market entirely.

In Britain, a new law will wipe out degrees from public funded universities in areas of alternative medicine. This includes homeopathy and naturopathy. German and British medical insurance providers are also in the process of removing alternative therapies from reimbursements.

In Australia, more than 400 doctors, researchers, and scientists have allied to lobby universities to close down alternative medical degrees. They have directed their venom at chiropractic, but it also includes traditional Chinese herbal medicine, homeopathy, naturopathy, reflexology, and aromatherapy. They are calling these "quackery" and touting "evidence-based medicine" and the "scientific rigor" process. They demand the government cease reimbursing for alternative care.

On the home front, the FDA just admitted in court documents that the agency "wants to protect the market for FDA-approved drugs." Hello!! That's another way of saying "wants to protect the market for "big pharma" chemicals." Where does the FDA get the authority to protect the market for chemicals it approves? I've read the Food and Drug and Cosmetic Act. Such authority does NOT exist!

The FDA has now openly exposed its evil agenda. This is a new self-generated expansion of its legal authority since the agency, in its paperwork, failed to cite any legal precedent for their newfound position.

Oh, but it's even worse than that. The FDA has drafted new guidelines to regulate the very supplements you take. But, agencies and courts are required to consider the "intent" of the legislature in the bills that are enacted. You might remember, after a hard-fought war, Congress passed DSHEA in 1944. Called the Dietary Supplement Health and Education Act, it protected nutritional supplements from the government thugs. Now, 17 years later, the FDA is reinventing the "intent" of the legislation on its own, in an effort to spin its strangulating web around supplements.

In an attempt to reign in the FDA, the drafters of DSHEA, Senators Orrin Hatch and Tom Harkin, recently went to the FDA to tell them the intent from the law's original authors. What could be more accurate than the intent of drafters of DSHEA, right? Well, I just got a message from the Alliance for Natural Health that the FDA has snubbed the two senators by refusing to reconsider its interpretation of the law in light of the Senators' intent.

Friend, I have led the quest for medical freedom since 1990. We've won some important battles. But the war rages on. The most important is always the final battle. And, that one is up to you.

I don't want to dismantle "big pharma". I want a level playing field—a free market, where the best therapy can win. Not the current rigged system promoted, aided, and abetted by the "Fraud and Deception Administration."

If you want real change, you need to storm their offices with calls and letters demanding an end to the pervasive corporate presence in government and complete restoration of a totally free market. The most important medical tipping point in the U.S. today is your right to supplements rather than force-fed petrochemicals. You also have in inherent right to a level playing field in the food arena. That is, GMO "foods" should be so labeled. But, industry has that bottled up too.

It's an election year. Any candidate that has taken a contribution from "big pharma," Monsanto, or a similar entity should be shown the exit door. You need to tell them that! That's the only way we will reset the path of America to protect its people, and not the multinational corporations. Please join the Alliance for Natural Health at www.anh-usa.org. You'll get ongoing current updates. Medical freedom is not up to me. It's also up to you! Please join me in this work-in-progress by contacting your representatives today (you can find their contact information at www.usa.gov/Contact/Elected.shtml).

Ref: Brisbane Times Jan 26, 2012; Alliance for Natural Health 1-31-12

Looking for an Integrative physician near you? These organizations can help:
* American Board of Clinical Metal Toxicology—For a free list, www.abemt.org
* International College of Integrative Medicine—www.icimed.com
* American College for Advancement in Medicine—800-532-3688 or www.acam.org.

Ending the pharmaceutical companies, FDA, AMA, FTA and the government's control over our lives and keeping the God-given, natural cures for ourselves is up to *us*! Let our voices be heard loud and clear!

---

[1] "The Douglass Report" by Dr. William Campell Douglass II, MD September 2011 Volume II No 5 Page 6-7 "Defeating Floride—One Community at a time"
[2] "The Douglass Report" by Dr. William Campell Douglass II, MD July 2011, Volume II No 3
[3] ?????
[4] "The Best of the Douglass Report" by Dr. William Campbell Douglass, II, M.D. Volume VII Used by Permission.????? Date and time of permission or email/letter received
[5] http://www.military-biodefensevaccines.org/documents/articles/20021126.pdf

[6]   http://en.wikipedia.org/wiki/Epidemiology_of_autism

[7]   http://www.cdc.gov/ncbddd/autism/data.html

[8]   Personal phone call on 9/10/2012 from Tim at Advanced Bionutritionals who gave us permission if we copied it verbatim.

[9]   Personal phone call on 9/12/2012 where they gave us permission if we copied it verbatim.

Chapter Eleven

CUTTING OFF THEIR NOSE TO SPITE THEIR FACE OR SHOOTING THEMSELVES IN THE FOOT!

Do these filthy rich pharmaceutical companies, medical schools, and our government really believe they are exempt from all the diseases, illnesses and deaths to which we ordinary citizens succumb? Or could they possibly think that the drugs they concoct will actually cure them when they know they haven't been able to cure the general population?

Insanity, according to Einstein, is doing the same thing over and over but expecting different results. How naive can they be? How stupid do they think the public is?

I'm sure the pharmaceutical companies know by now that they are not immune from cancer, diabetes, hepatitis, encephalitis, influenza, rabies, tetanus, malaria, and other diseases—the list is endless.

I received the Spring 2011 issue of the, *Diet and Health Study News* announcing "with great sadness" the death of A.S. Schatzkin, PhD, principal investigator of the NIA-AARP Diet and Health Study, on January 20, 2011. They said he was "an internationally renowned expert in the field of nutrition and cancer." And what was the cause of his death? Cancer! One of his studies was a four-year randomized trial regarding a low fat, high-fiber diet. A doctor who studied cancer and then died of cancer? Something here doesn't quite add up, except the low-fat diet portion. Remember the low-fat diet was based on a theory that was never proven, but people with a high fat and natural foods diet have been proven to live a far healthier existence!

And yet, the pharmaceutical companies not only refuse to listen to anyone about the natural, God-given cures that are available and proven to heal, they will do whatever they can to stop the information from getting out and will stop anyone that tries to promote them!

Some of these people need these natural, God-given cures of nutrition, herbs, vitamins, and minerals if they want to stay healthy and live a longer, healthier, and happier life!

The FDA and the pharmaceutical industry have even managed to get laws passed to stop any good information from coming out on real cures. They have taken away the licenses of many doctors who have used natural cures rather than drugs. Some have even been jailed. This is a crime and the pharmaceutical industry, the FDA, the AMA, and the FTA should be punished. Actually some are being punished by taking some of their own concocted drugs and suffering the dangerous side effects, including death!)

This is not a comforting thought! I do wish (and at this time can only be a wish) that everyone could have the advantage of proven natural cures that are without any side effects.

If it is difficult for you to believe the strong hold and powers that "big pharma" has, just ask someone in a health food store what you should buy to cure anything. They aren't allowed to tell you. They may say one of their customers has used a particular substance and seemed to have some favorable results, for example. They can't say "cured" or recommend any particular herb, vitamin, mineral, or nutritional product for a specific ailment!

Remember, the vitamin, herb, and mineral companies are not allowed to print on the labels what these good these "foods" will accomplish! They can do so only if they pay the horrendous fee for "approval" as mentioned in an earlier chapter.

Some doctors who have lost their licenses are writing health newsletters. They have to make a living, and this is probably what they know best and it is very important to them.

It is also possibly why the many health practitioners (they need to make a living, too) have not attempted to go after the FDA, pharmaceutical companies, medical schools, and the government for the problems that all of these drugs are causing. This could end up being a very time consuming, costly, activity to attempt single-handedly.

Enough of us working together, however—writing our congressmen and women and whomever else has any authority or influence—and it certainly can be accomplished.

I learned recently that Senator Oren Hatch subscribes to at least one of the health newsletters that my husband and I receive. Perhaps, he might be a good person to start with. He probably knows of others in our government who are also interested in good health through nutrition, vitamins, minerals, herbs, and other natural cures.

Elizabeth Edwards (wife of former Senator John Edwards) would have liked to know there were cures for cancer. And she would probably still be alive today to see the mess John Edwards is in now. Many politicians' morals, in general, are disgusting and much of Hollywood isn't any better.

Pharmaceutical companies are even worse than Washington or Hollywood—they are willingly killing people. And in the long run, they are actually killing themselves. After all, they have a license to kill and our government even backs them up with protection from being sued!

Wake up, people! There *are* cures available for ailments that are considered "incurable."

We just need to know where to find these cures. Right now they lie with good, alternative doctors, chiropractors, health newsletters, and anywhere we can find good, natural-health knowledge. There is a lot of information out there on health that is purported to be good knowledge, but really isn't. We need to read enough about proven cures to be able to deduce what is good and what is not.

If you want to find an alternative doctor or integrative physician, there are a couple of organizations that may be of help:

International College of Integrative Medicine. www.icimed.com

American Board of Clinical Metal Toxicology. www.abemt.org

We need to get our medical schools that are training our doctors only in pharmaceuticals and surgery to incorporate natural cures with nutrition, vitamins, minerals, and herbs.

Might it help if the heads of the pharmaceutical companies, the FDA, and the AMA had to visit the hospitals that administer the chemotherapy and other treatments they have concocted and approved for "curing" cancer and other diseases? They also need to visit the wards to see how the children that are dying of cancer are doing and what their parents are going through!

To put it bluntly, their cures are a dead end! There could be plenty of good instructors in our medical schools to teach about nutrition, vitamins, minerals, and herbs. More and more of our doctors are becoming interested in becoming "alternative" Doctors, if they weren't afraid of losing their licenses. They could also use the doctors that have lost their licenses for using alternative methods.

There are the chiropractors with a lot of knowledge on good health through nutrition, vitamins, herbs, and minerals. (Chiropractors are fun to go to—they will crack you up!)

The Amish could be another source of information for instructors. Many of the Amish people are very knowledgeable on health and healing with herbs. They rarely visit medical doctors—They don't need to.

In polls, the people in this country report that they are most concerned about "the economy" or "jobs." Their response should be "our health." People should be concerned with the one-sided teaching in medical schools.

What good is the best job or all the money in the world if your life is at risk and you are dying? In other words, would you rather be wealthy or healthy? If Natural cures and nutrition were taught in medical schools, this country would be much healthier and we wouldn't need near the health insurance we "think" we need now. We might not get as healthy as the people in Okinawa, but we would certainly be much healthier than Americans are now. We would live longer, more active, and happier lives! Natural cures have been around for thousands of years, patented drugs are fairly new.

The money we would save on doctors, hospitals, medication, canes, walkers, wheelchairs, nursing homes, and home healthcare is significant. Just think of all the money our government could save, too. It would distribute much less money in Medicare and Medicaid expenses. We would need fewer hospitals, fewer nursing homes, and all the other government health service providers!

Consider all the jobs that would be lost if we didn't have need for all these things. The former medical industry workers could open more health food stores, because we will need more places to buy these good products! We will need more alternative doctors and chiropractors to go to if we do get ill or out of joint. How about more farmers to grow the good foods? Are the people that manufacture drugs, willingly killing us, and giving us debilitating side effects to line their pockets really worth being concerned about?) The Pharmaceutical Companies do NOT want you well! Why should they? They only make their money when you are ill and they can sell you their drugs! They are, after all, licensed to kill!

If we don't start doing something *now*, it's only going to get worse! Don't say, or even think, you will do something about this tomorrow because tomorrow never comes! Tomorrow is the day we talked about yesterday, which is today!

Mark Twain wrote, "When you are confronted with a difficult decision, do what is right. You will please a few and you will amaze the rest!" [1] We all have a conscience. It is there to guide us in the right direction, if we don't run away from it. It is past time to stop racing away and do what is right. Good, natural, proven cures can be just around the corner if we stop taking the wrong turns. You too, will be amazed at how good you will feel—all over!

Just do it!

We, *the people*, must take our government, our lives, and our health back!

---

[1]   http://www.ldschurchnews.com/articles/print/61134/Messages-of-inspiration-from-President-Monson.html

Dictionary

Simvastatin

Statin medicines

Federal Drug Administration—FDA

Federal Trade Commission—FTC

American Medical Association—AMA

Poison—Any substance which kills or injures when introduced into a living organism; that which has an evil influence on health or moral purity; having a deadly or injurious quality

References

Barefoot, Robert—"The Disease Conspiracy (The FDA Suppression of Cures)" printed by RGM Management LLC

Barefoot, Robert; Reich MD, Carl J, "The Calcium Factor: The Scientific Secret of Health and Youth" printed by Central Plains Book manufacturing Inc Web: www.cureamerica.net

Douglass, II M.D, Dr. William Campbell.—The Douglass Report, and Newsletters on natural healing. Address: The Douglas Report, (Real Health News from Medicine's Most Notorious Myth-Buster) 819 N. Charles St., Baltimore, MD 21201. Phone: 603-236-4633 (9 t0 6 EST) Web: www.DouglasReport.com

Health Central Hospital—10000 West Colonial Drive Ocoee, FL 34761 (407) 296-1000

HSI—Health Sciences Institute 819 N. Charles Street, Baltimore, MD 21201. eMail: health@pubsvs.com. Phone: 915-849-4607 Fax: 410-230-1273

The Inquisitor—http://www.inquisitr.com/142881/drug-use-now-kills-more-people-than-traffic-accidents-study/

Klenner DR, Frederic R., http://www.doctoryourself.com/klennerbio.html

Levy MD, JD, Thomas E.—his books, *Curing the Incurable—Vitamin C, Infectious Diseases, and Toxins*, with over 1,200 Scientific References and *Stop America's #1 Killer!*.

WXYZ-TV Channel 7, 20777 W. 10 Mile Rd., Southfield, MI 48075-1086, http://www.wxyz.com

Pauling, Linus and Cameron E.—Cancer and Vitamin C: A Discussion of the Nature, Causes, Prevention, and Treatment of Cancer With Special Reference to the Value of Vitamin C (Camino Books) ISBN 0-940159-21-X

Pinkus MD, Dr. Michael—Dr. Newton's—Books and CD's, (Healing ourselves) Address: Dr. Newton's, 60 York street, Portland, ME 04101

Rowens, Dr. Robert J.—Second Opinion, Healing Volume, (Natures Cures) Address: Second Opinion, P.O. Box 8051, Norcross, GA 30091-8051 Phone: 800-262-3164 or 770-399-5617 Web: www.secondopinionnewsletter.com

Sinatra MD, Dr. Stephen—Booklets, etc. (Nutrition and Natural Health), Address: Advanced BioSolutions, P.O. Box 3277, Lancaster, PA 17604. Phone: 800-304-1708

Taubes, Gary—"Why We Get Fat and What to Do About It" (Random House Digital)

Whitaker MD, Dr. Julian—"Reversing Heart Disease" (Warner Books) ISBN 0-446-67657-8, "Reversing Hypertension" (Warner Books) ISBN 0-446-52286-4

Williams, Dr. David G.—"The World Atlas of Alternatives", "Unabridged Library Of Medical Lies" drdavidwilliams.com Phone: 1-800-527-3044

Wright, MD. Dr. Jonathon V.—"Library of Food and Vitamin Cures" P.O. Box 925, Frederic, MD 21705